Beauty and the Breast

Beauty *and the* Breast

A TALE OF BREAST CANCER, LOVE, AND FRIENDSHIP

MERRILL JOAN GERBER

coffeetownpress

Seattle, WA

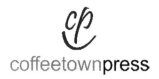

coffeetownpress

Coffeetown Press
PO Box 70515
Seattle, WA 98127

For more information go to: www.coffeetownpress.com
www.merrilljoangerber.com

This book is not a substitute or meant to be consulted for professional medical, legal, or financial advice. The author has presented her story. Names and identifying details have been changed, except when used by permission. You are encouraged to seek the advice of medical professionals if you have medical questions or concerns.

Cover design by Sabrina Sun
Beauty and the Breast

ISBN: 978-1-60381-526-0 (Trade Paper)
ISBN: 978-1-60381-574-1 (eBook)

Library of Congress Control Number: 2016942822

Printed in the United States of America
10 9 8 7 6 5 4 3 2 1

PRAISE FOR
BEAUTY AND THE BREAST

"An intimate, touching, moving portrait of the self in peril and in pain, written with characteristic intelligence & lucidity by Merrill Joan Gerber."
>—Joyce Carol Oates, author of *Soul at the White Heat* and winner of the National Humanities Award

"Short, easily digestible chapters. [Gerber] also includes clear, black-and-white close-ups of her affected breast during various stages of treatment, among other images.... The featured photographs of the author make this one stand out among the pack."
>—*Library Journal*

"I LOVE IT!! I could not put it down. Merrill Joan Gerber tells the story without a drop of feeling sorry for herself. She never loses her sense of humor. I've read a lot of breast cancer books, but hers is so fresh, so endearing, there's nothing else like it."
>—Judy Blume, author of *Are you There, God? It's Me, Margaret,* and *In the Unlikely Event*

"I read *Beauty and the Breast* nonstop: the pages turn themselves. Horror, humor, humaneness, fear, fatigue, love, honesty, bravery, and so much more, including even charm—all movingly mingled. The book (science and sensibility) is the triumph of an ordeal overcome and transcended."
>—Cynthia Ozick, author of *Critics, Monsters, Fanatics, and other Literary Essays*

"Merrill Joan Gerber is one of the finest writers of our time. There is no way to stop reading this very moving, compelling, sad but affirmative memoir. Whatever she touches, she illuminates."
>—David Evanier, author of *Woody: The Biography*

"As much rumination on the mortal predicament as it is testament to the continuous discovery that is life, Merrill Joan Gerber's memoir of her negotiations with cancer makes for richly provocative reading. And in the hands of a gifted and insightful writer with a penchant for the humorously quotidian,

those negotiations are at once profound and entirely accessible. Cancer demands courage. Writing about it may require something like meta-courage."
—Lynn Stegner, author of *For All the Obvious Reasons*

"With fluid writing and pitch-perfect timing, Merrill Joan Gerber has written a remarkable story of a woman's breast cancer journey. The photos and paintings rendered by the author of her treatments, her doctors, her husband and children add a wonderful visual layer to the tale. The author draws a heartwarming picture of family and friends who stay at her side and from whom she draws comfort, hope and delight. Gerber shares humorous takes on much that goes awry and offers many moments of wonder, joy and gratitude as well."
—Nancy Levinson, author of *Moments of Dawn, an Alzheimer's Memoir* and a two-time breast cancer survivor

"*Beauty and the Breast* will pour into a reader just as it poured from the author into her keyboard. It is hard to break away. Her voice is so powerful and intimate… she has borne witness in a voice that is unique and yet will reach everyone who reads it just where they are in their own lives. A beautiful and irresistible book."
—Charlotte Zoe Walker, author of *Condor and Hummingbird* and winner of an O. Henry Award

"While reading *Beauty and the Breast*, I am close to tears all the time. Merrill's incredible clarity and honesty is profound and necessary. The details, the photographs, the emotions make me feel as if it's me going through this. It's a real page-turner."
—Mary Trunk, documentary film maker (Merrill Joan Gerber is one of four women artists in her film, *Lost in Living*)

"*Beauty and the Breast* could be one of those books like Dr. Spock's Baby and Child Care that just doesn't quit selling because there is always another group that needs to know. The voice throughout the narrative is so superb. In some ways, the book feels more like a novel than a memoir. The pictures are extremely, extremely important. The interesting thing is that, at the end, the book becomes less about breast cancer and escaping death as it is about mortality and the seasons of life."
—Dr. Dean Paschal, Emergency Room physician, New Orleans

"*Beauty and the Breast* has such a wonderful combination of humor, love of life, and sheer terror. It's about breast cancer, but so much more. And it is about a long and happy marriage and the cancer that doesn't interrupt it. Bravo!"
—Dr. Madeleine Moskowitz, Doctor of Psychology and breast cancer survivor

With appreciation and gratitude to the
Cancer Support Community, Pasadena

For my beloved friends in the watercolor painting class

And to the memory of Elena, Peggy and Amy

CONTENTS

ACKNOWLEDGMENTS

MY THANKS TO THE CHILDREN OF Martha Schrage Widawer, Michelle, Marla, and Mark, for permission to use their mother's Miami Beach high school collage photo. My thanks to Joel Martin, who designed the collage, for permission to use it.

My thanks to Laura Wending of the Cancer Support Community Pasadena for permission to use the image of the "circle of friends."

My thanks to Sarah Whipple for permission to use the memorial collage photo of her sister.

My thanks to Dr. Debbie Bracamonte, my oncologist, for permission to use her image.

My thanks to Cristina Mateo, my chemo nurse, for permission to use her image.

Thanks to the Personal Care Products Council Foundation for permission to use the "Look Good, Feel Better" image. Note that my photo of the" Look Good, Feel Better" purse was taken in 2011. It has been redesigned and updated since then.

My thanks to Peg Schulte, whose blog is the source of the "Cancer Card" image in Chapter Eleven. Check out www.pegoleg. com, where you'll find "Playing the Cancer Card" and lots of other interesting and relevant posts. She is working on her own book, *A Guide to Playing the Cancer Card.*

My thanks to Darlene Traxler, President of the Sierra Madre Pioneer Cemetery for permission to use the photo taken in the cemetery.

My thanks to Dr. Grace Fu, my primary care doctor.

My thanks Dr. Timothy Cotter, my cardiologist.

And finally, my appreciation and gratitude to the organization of Kaiser Permanente, and to all my doctors, nurses and techs, for their support, encouragement, superb medical skills and tireless care.

ONE
BREASTS ARE EVERYWHERE IN BROOKLYN

A TRIO OF BUXOM ITALIAN SISTERS WHO live next door to us in Brooklyn offer to help me sew my eighth-grade graduation dress. My mother knows nothing about sewing and the rule is that I have to make my own dress. Otherwise I can't graduate. I won't get credit for Home Ec (which is half cooking, half sewing). The cooking half is easy—grilled cheese sandwiches and chocolate pudding. But sewing a whole dress?

My mother and I buy white organdy material, yards of it. We buy the pattern that seems simple and pretty, and we buy things with which we need to sew: silver needles, white thread, lace and satin trim, and a zipper. We beg the Ianello sisters to help us get through this.

At the Ianello house, there is noise and laughter and the smell of spaghetti sauce cooking. All the sisters have huge breasts, and when they bend over the dining room table, their flesh shifts like the tides; their breasts swing and surge and flow like a dance within a dance. They have a life of their own.

I am fascinated by this; I am entranced. I imagine how sweet it would feel to lay my head against their breasts. My mother has nothing that ever pillowed me in this way. I am going to have nothing, just little stubs that have just begun to grow, but not very fast and without much confidence.

My grandmother, with whom we live, has soft shifting breasts. Two girls in my eighth-grade class have enormous breasts; the boys circle around them like Indians in a cowboy movie about to invade a fort. I already know there are two kinds of women— those beautifully endowed, and those like me.

Over a period of weeks, the dress takes shape. I have fittings. The Ianello sisters have me stand up on their dining-room table so they can pin an even hem, allowing my organdy dress to swing beautifully around my legs as I go up to the stage to get my diploma. The dress has lovely darts converging to points that my nipples should fill ... but they don't come anywhere near.

On the day of graduation at the Kingsway Theater on Kings Highway near my school, P.S. 238, I come to a decision in the darkness of the theater, as I sit in the second row (my last name starts with a G, meaning I will be called up soon). I will stuff tissues down the front of my new dress. I have tissues in a little white purse beaded with pearls, given to me by my aunt as a present. I bend forward in the dimness of the theater and push the tissues into the bosom of my dress to reach to the points of the darts. My plan is not well thought out. I wonder what will hold them in place, what will make them point the right way.

The principal is calling out the name of my classmate, "Rochelle Amateau," and then he calls "Doris Amerling," "Avram Bain," "Kim Bak Hong" (the Korean boy), and "Sheldon Finkleman." Suddenly he is at the G's, and I hear my name—"Merrill Joan Gerber." As I stand up, I feel the tissues shimmy past my chest, down past my waist, and fall like clumps of snowflakes along my thighs and onto the theater floor. I let them fall, stepping over them and kicking them to the side. I go up to the stage, my head bowed, my cheeks flaming with humiliation, to get my diploma. I graduate eighth grade.

Afterward, I go home with my family and pose for a picture on the grass in the front garden, in front of the bush of blue popcorn ball flowers. This is me, on graduation day in 1951. The address of my house is 405, the bench is where my grandmother used to sit every day. Spotty is the name of my dog.

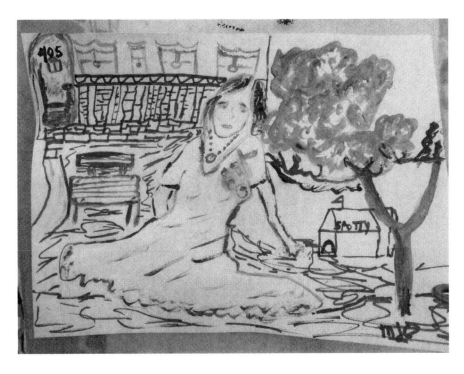

Merrill on grass under tree

TWO
THE DREADED LUMP APPEARS

A HUNDRED YEARS HAVE PASSED SINCE MY eighth-grade graduation. Somehow I have managed to seduce into my life what breasts are meant to elicit: beauty and boys and love and sex and eventually babies. I have nursed three beautiful daughters. My breasts have never come close to the endowments of the Ianello sisters, but I offered the world (my husband, my children) a facsimile, an authentic set of miniatures. When I was a teenager in the fifties, a crisis occurred having to do with my breasts. I was dating a young man, who at the beach one night under a full moon, tried to put his hand down the front of my square-cut summer dress.

"Mine?" he said.

"No! *Of course not!*"

He seemed to take this as permission and continued his foray into my camisole. He touched my breast.

"What are you *doing*!" I cried.

"Well, I asked you if you would mind and you said no."

"Would I *mind*? I thought you were asking 'Mine! Are these mine!' Of course they're not yours."

A simple semantic matter changed our world that night. I loved having him touch my breast. Both of them. I let him do it again and again. Night after night. Week after week. Reader, I married him.

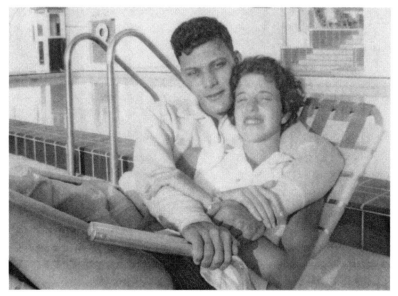

Reader, I married him

However, the storms of time have blown us along. My little girls have their own breasts and husbands and children. My beloved and I have bought an adjustable king-sized bed on which we change the angles of our limbs and watch old movies on TV. Now and then he reaches over and strokes my thigh. I never know what this signal implies (if anything). Is it an invitation, or is it like someone patting a dog to assure him he still belongs here as a member of this household? I sometimes pat him back, and that seems to complete the exchange.

One day, or one night, I find the dreaded lump in my breast. Who knows how I find it, who can remember? It's nothing, of course. Probably just a cyst. I've had many cysts. It's only eight months since my last mammogram. Surely there's nothing to worry about.

It's nothing. It will go away. Cysts come and go. No one in my family has had breast cancer—not my mother, my aunts, my grandmothers. They all had horrific strokes, and then lived ten years more—all of them—paralyzed, helpless, my mother on a feeding tube. But not a drop of breast cancer in my family. Other cancer, yes, but only a few cases. My father contracted leukemia, which hit him at fifty-five and killed him within three months.

But this lump, much smaller than a marble, is without a doubt *nothing*.

However, I seem to check it ten times a day. No matter how often I check it, it doesn't change, and it doesn't go away.

I finally make an appointment to see my doctor—a tall, beautiful Chinese woman, the age of one of my daughters. She is totally competent, unsentimental. "We all have to die, you know," she said at an earlier visit when I expressed fear about the losses that come with getting old. "Indeed, we all have to die." She smiled with such sweet reassurance, it seemed a pleasure to hear the news.

She feels the lump. Her fingertips listen, her eyes are off in space, but she feels deeply. Her touch is feather-light, then her fingers roll hither and thither, up and down, under and over.

"It's probably just a cyst," she says, but she makes a phone call and schedules an appointment for me for a STAT mammogram and ultrasound.

When I get home, I make dinner and say to my husband, "It's probably just a cyst." He nods and chews my special recipe of chicken thighs breaded with crushed Rice Krispies. We have chocolate pudding for dessert—my favorite comfort food—and I put whipped cream on it, shot from a can.

THE MAMMOGRAM ROUTINE IS TOTALLY FAMILIAR. I've done this for at least twenty-five years. Each breast gets slapped on a cold white shelf with the tech shoving and pulling it and then squashing it under the upper plate, turning the wheel and saying, "Hold your breath, don't breathe."

On this day, there is a new young tech who doesn't know when to stop twisting the black knob. "Hey! That's too much. Way too tight!"

"Sorry, my bad," she says.

Her bad?

In another room she checks the films—is it taking longer than usual this time?—and then returns, making no eye contact with me. She hands me the films in a rigid folder and instructs me to take them to the ultrasound department. "Do you need a chaperone?" she asks. She can guide me.

"No thanks." Does she fear I will switch these for some better mammogram films? Does she think I will steal them and sell them on a street corner? I go speeding through the familiar halls with my husband at my side. I am already thinking we will stop at Food For Less on the way home and get some fish for dinner. Chicken and fish are what we mostly eat now. And plant-based foods. We've given up red meat. For our health's sake. Given up foods that could cause cancer.

AS A RESULT OF MY MANY lengthy and boring tests in this medical facility, I have, over the years, purely for entertainment, developed a few thrilling sexual fantasies about being touched and handled in a dim room by a gentle nurse. The echo-cardiogram setting for my heart exam easily lends itself to this fantasy, as does the ultrasound breast exam. A cold gel is involved in both, a wand held by a caring woman dressed in white, some cautions as to "this will feel cold at first," and then the quiet privacy of our intercourse, our intimacy. In the case of the echo exam, I have been privy to glimpsing the red blood of my heart beating on the screen and have been able to hear the whoosh-thump of my valves opening and closing.

During the breast ultrasound, I feel the wand wandering over my breast while the tech, with her free hand, enters secret information on her keyboard. On the screen I see the landscape of my breasts—the craters of the moon, the jagged edges of outer space.

This time the ultrasound is taking a very long time. My husband is in the waiting room; he must be wondering at the delay. The wand rests too long on my left breast. It repeats itself, it starts over, it presses too hard, it hurts. I look at the tech but read in the woman's face a dire warning: "Don't ask me a thing. Don't even try." Today there is nothing sexy about this scenario. Nothing!

"Will someone tell me something? *Eventually?*"

The tech rises from her chair and hands me a towel to wipe the gel off my breast. She's finished. She's only doing the one breast, the one with the lump. She leaves the room. I am cold all over. I am freezing. I have a blouse, I have a sweater there on the chair. I put them both on. I peek at the screen of the monitor and see my name printed there. I see in detail more of the lunar landscape of my breast: craters and ridges, black holes.

No one can stop me from taking a picture of this—I always have my camera in my purse, and there's no one here to disapprove. Click, click … the moonscape is mine. All those circles and jagged holes, all those (please God) mere cysts. But should a room where women are required to be nearly naked be kept this cold?

A man suddenly comes into the room, followed by the tech. This man is the real thing, the authority, a doctor—the kind in a white coat, with his name embroidered over his pocket.

"We hate to tell a woman a thing like this," he says. Of course, my soul knows what is coming. I lean against the gurney on which I was so recently supine. "This is what we see when we see cancer."

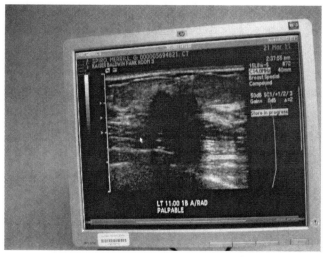

"This is what we see when we see cancer."

He points at the black hole. What I see is a beast. My breast is the *Beauty* and this sinister black eye is *the Beast*.

"Do you see these irregular edges?" he says, not expecting an answer. "It's not too large, however. Under two centimeters."

Is that good or bad, it being under two centimeters? How big is a centimeter? Why didn't I listen in math class when I was ten years old? Why don't they use regular English words that have meaning—inches, or marbles. No bigger than a marble. Why do I have ragged edges in my breast? Who gnawed away at that perfect circle of a cyst?

However, I am no longer whoever I was before I got this news. The old Merrill is not the present Merrill. My teeth begin to chatter. There is the cold of death in this room.

"Of course, we can't be sure until a biopsy is taken," the doctor says. "Could you come in tomorrow to have a biopsy?"

"Someone call my husband, please," I say. "Call him. His name is Joe; he's in the waiting room."

I am shaking with tremendous chills. I can hear my teeth hitting one another like jackhammers. The tech puts a cotton blanket around my shoulders. "Here, sit down," she says. Some others have come into the room. A nurse arrives with my husband.

"I have cancer," I say. He takes my hand. He's not the Joe he used to be either. We are sliding on black ice straight down a steep mountain; we are about to crash and burn.

The doctor in white leads Joe to the screen and points out some critical features of the black hole.

"Can you come back tomorrow?" the doctor asks again.

Someone else says, "What about today? She's here now … why can't we do it today?" I could kiss her, whoever she is. *Let's hurry this along. Otherwise it could be a long, terrible ordeal.*

I agree. Yes, I'm here today; I want them to notice. I say it loudly. "I'm here right now."

"We'll do the biopsy today then." Preparations are made. I am led back to lie flat on the gurney. I am again divested of my blouse and my sweater. Something cold is painted over my breast.

A female doctor arrives. She is all Competent Woman—blonde,

pretty, with lively round breasts, a sweet smile. She's gorgeous and perfect. I wish my daughters had gone to med school.

"We'll numb your breast. We'll put in a marker. We'll take six little snips of tissue. You'll hardly feel it."

"Go right ahead." The new Merrill can be generous with snips of tissue, rotten tissue, poisonous tissue. Who needs it? And they do go right ahead. Here comes the long needle. I don't look. The doctor just stabs it deep inside my body. The needle moves around, it comes out, it goes in again. Something icy is sprayed on my breast. *Snip, snip, snip, snip, snip, snip.*

"All done." A nurse sits me up, presses an ice pack against my breast. She wraps an elastic bandage tightly around my chest, around both breasts, and we're all done. "Go home now and rest."

That's it?

My husband and I stumble outside into the sunlight. We find where Joe parked the car and he begins to drive us home. Nothing is said about stopping at Food For Less. Joe might be saying something to me, but I can't hear him above the chattering of my teeth.

I'm dead, I think. What about that? After so long a time of being Merrill, Merrill is going to be dead.

"But wait," I say. "We have no bananas."

"We have no bananas today," he repeats. Is this a joke?

"We have to stop at Dogwood's. It won't take long. I can't be without bananas. And I have to call Becky."

There's the rub. The children must be told. The mother must tell her daughters that they are now the issue of a first-degree relative with cancer. This will ruin their day. This could be their death sentence. How does a mother do this to them? How does she ensnare them in a genetic nightmare that sizzles with the threat of cancer?

For one thing, I remember that my cell phone almost never gets a signal, wherever I am. This may be my way out. I open my cell phone and there are two pathetic bars visible on the screen. I call Becky, my one daughter who lives nearby. The others are far away, hundreds of miles. This child is only two miles away. She must be warned first. She is the oldest.

"It's Mom," I say, when she answers the phone.

"Where are you?"

"We're in the car, going to Dogwood's for bananas."

"But did you have the ultrasound?"

"Oh yes, I did."

"And …?"

"And they sort of see something in there. Something sort of maybe like cancer."

"Oh Mom! Oh Mom!"

"It's small. Less than two centimeters." She will know what a centimeter is. She has advanced degrees, a good education. "They took a biopsy. I feel fine. There was nothing to it."

"Oh Mom," she says again.

"Remember when you had a lump and they thought it was cancer, but then it was nothing?"

"That was almost twenty years ago."

"Did I ever tell you I called that radio psychologist, Dr. Viscott? I was so scared that you might die that I was in a panic. I heard him on the radio one day and called him and I told him I was so worried about you I couldn't bear it."

"I didn't know you called a radio psychologist. What did he say?"

"He said I was a narcissist. The bastard. He said I was thinking only of myself."

There is silence on the phone. Outer space swallows Becky's comment.

"We're breaking up. I'll talk to you later, Becky. I have no signal here."

"Okay, Mom."

"There, I did it," I tell my husband. "One daughter down, two to go. And then I'll tell my sister. How am I doing?"

"Fine," he says. "But you don't have to do everything this minute. Maybe we should go home. You need to rest. Do we have to stop at Dogwood's?"

"I need halvah," I tell him, "chocolate-covered halvah."

DOGWOOD'S IS A TINY ARMENIAN PLACE that sells oddly shaped vegetables, long skinny sweet potatoes or enormous five-pound sweet potatoes. They sell mysterious eastern grains and nuts, ten pound containers of olive oil from Greece. Everything is very inexpensive. We sometimes buy home-cooked food made by the owner, Armenian soup with chicken legs and bulgur in it.

I don't know why I want to be in here. I'm sick. I'm dizzy. A headache has engulfed me. I come here all the time and never before have I been dying while I'm here. How do they sell cilantro for so little, twenty-five cents a bunch? Onions, two dollars for ten pounds. What's wrong with those onions? I am lost in a reverie of vegetables, wandering the aisles, touching enormous tomatoes, stroking stalks of fennel. The olives here, in big bins, in black salty brine, are enticing. My father loved them "from the old country." He called them *mislinnas*. He died of leukemia at a young age. Fifty-six. I can't even tell him I now have cancer. Why isn't he here to take care of me? When I was a little girl, in Brooklyn, on cold winter nights he would heat a frying pan on the stove and warm my bed sheets with it. Where is my father? Where do the dead *go*?

"Bananas," my husband reminds me, "and then let's leave."

When I get to the banana bin, a woman who seems delighted to see me, a beautiful woman, approaches me with open arms and embraces me.

"Mom!" she says. "I'm so happy I found you here."

"Becky," I say. "I'm sorry. I didn't intend this. I love you so much. I hated to have to tell you this news."

"You'll be fine," she says. "We'll all take care of you. Don't worry, Mom."

We load up on bananas, on Brussels sprouts. At least we won't starve.

Becky wanders away and then surprises me with two bars of chocolate-covered halvah with the word *Joyva* on the wrapper. They knew this food was about joy when they named it. The man who named it was a Jewish guy from Brooklyn. I always knew this.

He and I were meant for each other. We should have married. If I die soon, however, I will die drugged by the beauty of chocolate and I will die happy.

THREE
THE BIOPSY REPORT

THIS IS WHAT MY BREAST LOOKS like the day after the biopsy: a little pink bruise, a little Band-Aid strip, and I'm back at the helm of my life. Maybe that's enough, maybe that's all we have to do. All the rest has been a big mistake, imagining that the lump was cancer. Not in my family! We women die of stroke. It's our policy, our destiny.

You can't presume one has cancer without a biopsy. And no one has called me yet to tell me bad news. I may get away scot-free. I may just go back to making a shopping list for Food For Less.

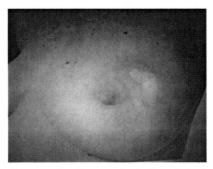

Breast after biopsy, little Band-Aid

But then, three days later, I get a call from the nurse of the doctor who did the biopsy—she has the official results. She reads the report to me. It all sounds like gibberish. I tell her so.

"When you see the surgeon, she will explain all the details."

"But is it cancer?"

"I'm afraid so. Yes, dear, it is cancer."

I ask that the report be emailed to me, and this is what appears on the screen.

This is what an official report of cancer looks like. Feel free to bypass it.

March 21 2011

Guided needle core biopsy

Invasive mammary carcinoma with ductal and lobular features

Histological grade: moderately differentiated (Nottingham Composite Grade 2 out of 3)

Tubule formation: score 3 out of 3

Mitotic Count: score 1 out of 3

Composite Score: 7 out of 9

Small focus suggestive of high grade ductal carcinoma in situ. Unfavorable.

Tumor size: 1.7 greatest diameter measured from microscopic slides

Estrogen and progesterone receptor Status (invasive tumor and DCIS: both negative)

No definite lymphovascular invasion identified

Focal Benign Ductal hyperplasia

No microcalcifcations or perineural invasion identified.

Microscopic Description:

Sections which have been cut at multiple levels show an invasive mammary carcinoma with features of infiltrating ductal carcinoma and invasive lobular carcinoma .

The tumor is composed of irregular solid nests of cells infiltrating stroma showing desmoplasia and hyalinization. The tumor cells show large pleomorphic nuclei with finely granular chromatic and prominent single to multiple reddish nucleoli and abundant slightly basophilic staining cytoplasm. Up to four mitotic figures are identified in a count of ten high power fields.

Er and Pr results: negative, no tumor cells staining

Clinical history

Mass 1.7 cm

Calcifications: no

So that is what bad news looks like. "Prominent. Infiltrating. Invasive. Abundant. And what's that one awful word? *Unfavorable*? Is all the rest favorable? This can't be good. This can't be me because I feel so well. This can't be cancer.

A Rodgers & Hart melody suddenly comes to me and like a madwoman I begin to sing: "This can't be cancer, because I feel too well ...." In the original song, of course, the subject is "love." The singer laments that if it were love, she would surely be dizzy, sighing, and sobbing. And if I really had cancer, wouldn't I feel sick?

But it is cancer, Merrill. Get used to it.

FOUR
TELLING MY DAUGHTERS

A WARNING, DEAR READER: BELOW IS A photo of my breast taken just a few days after the biopsy. If you feel uneasy, just skip over it. The real violence to my breast has not even begun.

In fact, cancer is a messy business. It's so connected to our blood, our skin, the air we breathe—but let us hope it will never migrate to our bones, lungs or liver—also to our vanity, to our sense of being female and beautiful, of being sexy. This image of my breast, you can see at once, is not at all about sex, it is clearly not a model for a *Playboy* centerfold.

But powerless as I may be against cancer, I am ruthless with my camera in my journey toward discovery. I am the detective who must get to the truth, get to the facts, and if necessary, get real about facing the fear.

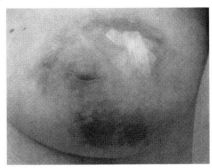

Breast three days after biopsy

My younger daughters may have been put on alert by Becky, for when I do reach them by phone? Each of them has some reassurance for me taken from the news or personal experience— each knows a friend who is doing well after her cancer diagnosis. Both these friends were teenagers when I knew them, but are now young mothers.

Mothers who now have breast cancer. Cancer is most aggressive in young women. One daughter's friend is Stage Four (the worst— there is no Stage Five). My other daughter's friend, though having a lower stage, has decided there are other threats she will not countenance. She will bypass all treatments but the knife. She has chosen to have a double mastectomy. Both breasts off. She will skip all the rest: chemo, radiation, and a lifetime of fear.

In turn, my children reassure me there are very good treatments now. I reassure them that now is the best time in history to be facing breast cancer. Not one of us really knows if we believe what we are saying.

I have had only my biopsy, not yet my surgery. What comes later will tell the bigger story. What is discovered afterward, in the cancerous tissue, will write the future. The story is only at its opening scene.

FIVE
THE BEAUTIFUL FACE OF MY SURGEON

T HE WHITE COAT, YES, THE NAME over her pocket, yes, Her face conveys confidence, tough intelligence, and her eyes shine with a warlike determination to fight what's in my breast. Over the years, she's had knowledge of my breasts. She's considered my cysts, my dense breast tissue, and she once treated me for an infection … making sure I came back in ten days so she could see for herself that the painful red place on my breast was gone.

This time we have a deadly serious subject to discuss. I've brought my old cassette recorder and a tape. (I have read that taping what the doctor tells you about your cancer treatment is a good idea, that you can't take it all in at once). I ask her permission. It's fine, she says, she doesn't mind.

"What I'm going to tell you is exactly the same thing I'd tell a doctor with breast cancer who came in to see me before surgery. I take nothing for granted; I will tell you every detail that I think you must know."

On a lit background my surgeon displays my mammogram films. These are the films from eight months ago.

"See," she says, "there's nothing unusual going on here." I have to take her word for this since all I can see are Van Gogh-like swirls in the black-and-white mystery on the screen. "This can happen. Mammograms do not find every cancer."

Why not? I want to ask. *Why have I been having these tests every year for decades?*

"Now," she says. "This is what I think. You're a good candidate for a lumpectomy. Let me see here …" and she has me lie back on the examining table. I haven't been given a gown, so I simply pull my sweater up over my breasts. She, like my GP, looks toward the wall or the ceiling—as she feels every tiny area of my breast.

"It's a small tumor." Now she is feeling under my arm, perhaps three or four inches away from where the lump resides in my left breast just above the nipple.

"I'll remove the sentinel lymph node," she explains. "If we find no cancer cells in it, we won't take any additional nodes, and then you won't have much danger of lymphedema. Just before surgery we'll inject a nuclear tracer and a blue dye into your bloodstream. These will illuminate the possible path of cancer cells. Your pee will be blue for a couple of days. If any of the cells have spread beyond your breast, the dye will show it."

I hear my cassette tape grinding along; it's getting all this. I'm already confused. I glance at Joe, but he hasn't much comprehension in his face. In fact, I see nothing but the same kind of confusion I feel. What are we doing here? Why is our life now going to be an endless series of trips to this medical center, why will I have to have a piece of my breast cut out, why should I have to worry that blue-colored cancer cells may have escaped into my lymph nodes? Didn't I cook us lots of broccoli? Didn't we often have peaches and cherries last summer? A few chocolate chip cookies could not have caused all this trouble? (Could they?)

She continues: "After the lumpectomy, you'll need radiation, but probably not chemo. Twenty-five percent of women need a second surgery to get clean margins. That means we won't know till we see the specimen we remove if we've gotten a good margin between the stained cancer cells and healthy tissue. I'll do my best to get it all, but you never know."

I'm thinking about statistics now, with my pathetic mathematical knowledge. I conclude that twenty-five out of a hundred women have to go back for a second surgery. One surgery seems more than enough to me.

"And," says the doctor after a pause, "twenty-five percent of women have the HER-2 neu factor. You don't want that."

"I don't?"

"Well, that would mean a full year of infusions with Herceptin. That would mean chemo every three weeks for a year. Herceptin is a relatively new monoclonal antibody that's been recently discovered to be successful in treating advanced breast cancer."

"Advanced?"

"Herceptin also seems to have good results with early stage cancer, which is what you have. You have Stage One cancer. But you also have Grade Three, which means you have some aggressive cells in there. They're fast-growing; they've grown so fast we see some dead tissue in your biopsy specimen as the cancer cells have overrun the healthy tissue."

I've heard enough. I hear the cassette tape click off. I know I should turn it over, but it seems pointless. Nothing it is recording will I ever want to play again, not in my lifetime.

"We know you're double-negative," my surgeon says, "that means your cancer is not estrogen or progesterone receptive, so we can't block its growth with the medicines we have to treat that. But if you're HER 2 neu positive, we do have Herceptin."

I'm thinking about the names of medicines. Herceptin must mean "her is intercepted"—why don't they call it "Sheceptin?" Why would I want to be intercepted? I'm so tired. I want to go home. The doctor is now telling Joe that my odds are good with a lumpectomy. Do we agree that I want a lumpectomy and not a mastectomy? With a mastectomy, I'd need no radiation treatments. "And of course, radiation means going to a radiation center every weekday for six weeks."

Every weekday for six weeks?

"Radiation treatment doesn't take very long," she says. "Maybe five minutes total in the LINAC—that's the linear accelerator. But for that you would have to go either to Ontario or to Los Angeles. We don't have a radiation facility here."

"Why not?" I say. But by now I've heard enough.

I definitely do not want a mastectomy. I am not ready to lop off a whole breast of mine. Let's just get this surgery over with; let's see what the blue dye says.

BEFORE WE LEAVE TODAY THERE'S JUST one more requirement. The surgery is set for a week from today. I am required to have a brief visit with an anesthetist in another department. The one assigned to me is a sweet young black woman. She has to tilt my head far back to see if it's flexible enough to allow intubation.

A tube has to be stuck down my throat. She also has to send me now to the lab for some blood tests required before surgery. I think of needles in my flesh again (I know that's really nothing, nothing at all) and my eyes well up with tears.

"Sweetheart," the anesthetist says to me, squeezing my shoulders, "this is not really a difficult surgery. It's quite superficial, and your surgeon is terrific. You won't have much pain. What's really terrible is this disease. And that's why you're here—to get it out and be rid of it."

SIX
THE BLISS OF NOTHINGNESS—
AND THEN THE KNIFE

WHAT IS THIS LITTLE PACKAGE THEY sent home with me? Aren't surgeons supposed to scrub up in the hospital before surgery? Now it seems the patients are being asked to do the scrubbing at home.

There are explicit instructions and a stern warning: "Using this product may cause serious and permanent eye injury if permitted to enter or remain in contact with the eye. If swallowed, contact a Poison Control Center right away."

The kit includes a sharp pick for cleaning under the nails, a scrub brush for "cleaning the cuticles and the interdigital spaces between the fingers," and a sponge saturated with "cocamide DEA, lauramine oxide, PEG-75, glucono-delta-lactone, hydroxyethylcellulose, and tridecyl alcohol."

"Shower and scrub with this kit at bedtime before your surgery and again two hours before you leave for the hospital. This will significantly reduce the number of microorganisms on the hands and forearms, or on the body, prior to surgery."

I am puzzled by these instructions. Let us imagine I go to bed at 11 p.m.— all scrubbed up and sterilized by the time I fall asleep (if I should so lucky as to fall asleep). My orders are to be at the hospital by 4 a.m., which means (considering the instructions for use of the sterilization kit) I am required to wake at 2 a.m., climb into the shower and decontaminate myself a second time. Do the powers-that-be who design these commands think that a patient about to go under the knife, in the hours she is in bed trying not to have a psychotic break, is going to have messy, wild, and steamy sex between shower one and shower two?

In any case, how will I be able to sleep? Surgery is a week away.

I appeal to my GP. She understands my plight; she agrees to prescribe a sleeping pill. I love the sight of it, a beautiful thing, a small pill that promises to get me out of here, get me to nowhere where I want to be, where fear does not live.

On the first night, I ingest it with gratitude. Within minutes, in fact within seconds, I feel myself disappearing. I can feel it happening in that instant between full consciousness and the awareness of the edges blurring, of the room expanding to a blissful white fog, and then … nothingness.

In the morning, I wake up full of good cheer. However, Joe tells me I have been mumbling during the night, speaking to ghosts, flinging my arms about, and hitting him smack in the face. He also says that at one point I picked up the bedside phone and began whispering words that sounded to him like phone sex.

I decide to look up my sleeping pill on the internet. I learn the following:

This drug is a sedative, also called a hypnotic. It affects chemicals in your brain that may become unbalanced and cause sleep problems (insomnia) rash; hives; itching; difficulty breathing; tightness in the chest; swelling of the hands, legs, mouth, face, lips, eyes, throat, or tongue; throat closing; unusual hoarseness; abnormal thinking; behavior changes; chest pain; confusion; decreased coordination; difficulty swallowing or breathing; fainting; fast or irregular heartbeat; hallucinations; memory problems (e.g., memory loss); mental or mood changes (e.g., aggression, agitation, anxiety); new or worsening depression; severe dizziness; shortness of breath; suicidal thoughts or actions; vision changes, violent behaviors.

This is not a complete list of all side effects that may occur. If you have questions about side effects, contact your health care provider. Call your doctor for medical advice about side effects.

I'm not daunted in the least by this. We've all seen the Lunesta butterfly sweetly fluttering about the happily sleeping beautiful woman. We've also seen the Ambien TV ad in which a crowing rooster terrifies the man who can't get to sleep. He is driven to near madness till Ambien wafts him into the heavenly, restful world of peace and beauty. Never mind that the voiceover babbles at extremely high speed about the possible side effects: night driving (followed by amnesia), having sex (followed by amnesia), cooking a meal (followed by amnesia), and even suicide (followed, of course, by permanent amnesia).

Side effects, as we know, happen on the side, not to everyone, not likely to me. Eating hot dogs can cause cancer, but does it happen to everyone?

(Did it happen to me? Perhaps it did. Who really knows?)

I take my sleeping pill every night till the night before surgery. I take my chances, but I have to sleep.

Still, there is the problem of getting through the daytime hours. Something makes me want to cry. A hard sharp wheel turns in my chest and seems to pump tears up to my eyes. I don't want Joe to see me cry so I go out into the backyard. I cry near the rosemary bush, near the orange tree, near the wisteria vine. I cry quietly, my tears falling on the yellow nasturtium blossoms. I have read you can eat nasturtium flowers, even the seeds. I am not hungry as I cry, and I absolutely don't want my neighbor, the woman who hates me, to hear me cry. She will know something is wrong, and she will rejoice. I don't want to hate her more than I already hate her because it will cause me stress, and stress, we all know, is bad for the immune system. When the immune system is stressed, cancer gets a free ride.

Still, I cry, and no longer softly. My desperate sobs alarm even me—and her dogs begin to bark. This is what the conflict is about:

her barking dogs and my begging her to quiet them. I will not let myself think about this endless quarrel now, since it will be very bad for me, but let me say this much. For years her three dogs barked for hours all day, and often during much of the night. When I told her we were unable to sleep, she simply said, "We like our dogs to bark. That's why we got them."

Before dawn on the morning of surgery, after I have sterilized all parts of my body (once, not twice), I develop a stomachache so intense that I fear I can't leave the house. Should there not be a toilet in every car? Think of the millions of people who commute and suddenly need a bathroom. There's relentless cramping in my gut. Fear can do that, can't it? Fear of a knife going into my breast this morning.

I won't be present to observe this. I have been assured that I will be in that other reality where an unconscious person temporarily confronts what death must be like on a permanent basis.

I get dressed and bejewel myself. The jewels I choose to wear, besides my wedding ring, are my mother's wedding ring and a four-leaf-clover necklace on a gold chain that my father gave me for good luck on my exams when I was in high school.

"Okay, Joe, I'm ready. Let's go." Of course, I am not permitted to have breakfast. Joe seems to be considering a bowl of brown oatmeal. Then he dumps it in the sink.

Why do they need us there at 4 a.m. when the surgeon does not arrive till 7 a.m.? This is a mystery to all of us in the waiting room, each awaiting his or her own surgeon. There's not much on TV at 4 a.m. though—a few people are checking their cell phones for messages. *Every one of us here has to go through with this,* I think. *There's no getting out of it.* I remember having that same thought when I arrived at the hospital each of the three times I gave birth. "Let's not do this," I said to Joe each time.

Today I don't give him any grief. He's so tired, it's so early, and he has such a long wait ahead of him. He looks so worried. A nurse comes to the waiting room and calls my name. Joe squeezes my hand as he relinquishes me. He's on his own now.

In the pre-surgery room, they give me a hospital gown, a high-tech garment that pumps warm air against my skin and comes with a remote control to create the ideal temperature. They put a pair of blue "bear paw" slippers on my feet. Then an IV needle is plunged into my arm.

After this, Joe is allowed to come back and sit with me. We are in a big room, and in every curtained cubicle there is a patient like me waiting for a surgeon like my surgeon. Someone who knows her business. Someone who is going to fix us up so we can go home and plant sunflower seeds.

"Let's grow lots of flowers this spring," I tell Joe. "Lots of tomato plants."

"I'll buy you a hundred tomato plants," Joe says, the most romantic thing he has ever said to me in his life.

A lovely woman, the black anesthetist I have met before, appears at the foot of my bed. "You'll be just fine," she says. "We'll take good care of you." She reaches for my hand (the one without the needle in it) and we hold hands for a moment. She says to Joe, "We'll take good care of her." I am so grateful I could cry. The nurse adds something to my IV and then begins to wheel me away from my husband. "I'll be perfectly fine," I assure him. Though I feel the buzz of fading light, I am awake long enough to see the long hall, the green-tiled operating room, and in it, what seems like a small army of men and women wearing cute little green hats. They are all smiling at me.

"You'll be fine," they say to me, one by one. "Just fine."

SEVEN
ARE YOU A TEN? SURVIVING SURGERY

"**T**AKE A DEEP BREATH. THAT'S GOOD. Can you open your eyes?"

I swim into light. There's the world again as I left it. A nurse, a cubicle, a slight weight on the left side of my chest.

"What are you? A five? A ten?"

"I would love to be a ten. But I don't think I could be. My husband's mother thought I wasn't pretty enough for her son. It's not likely I'm a ten. At best maybe a nine."

"A nine! You have that much pain?"

"Who's talking about pain?"

"How much pain are you in?"

"I'm not in pain. I'm fine."

Then I shift my body slightly. *Ooh! There it is in red flashing lights. Pain.*

"It's not bad," I reassure the nurse. I really don't want them to think me ungrateful. Here I am, alive. The handsome face of my husband appears above me.

He tells me it's already been two hours since my surgery was finished. He tells me the surgeon talked to him, that everything went well. Now I'm ready to go home.

The nurse is trying to get me into my clothes. I notice that both my wedding ring and my mother's wedding ring (one on each hand) are covered with tape. I feel for my four-leaf-clover, relieved it's still around my neck. My father wanted me to have good luck all my life. His horseshoe ring for luck didn't do him much good. I hope for better luck with my lucky four-leaf clover.

Now that I'm dressed, the nurse puts a round object in my hand. "Here are pills for pain, but don't take one till you get home and can eat something first."

Joe has disappeared. I am required to use the bathroom with a nurse at my side. Then I am bundled into a wheelchair and whisked outside of the hospital into the bright April sunshine, where the air is fresh. *I'm alive.* I love the sight of Joe's car, dusty, with a dent or two and clearly in need of a wash, pulling up to the curb.

The nurse helps me transfer into the car. I think of the day I had my third baby girl at Holy Angels Hospital, so long ago. When they sent me home, the nurse, standing under a statue of the Holy Mother, waved to me and said, "See you next year."

This time, there's no precious baby in my lap, only a burning in my breast. We drive toward the mountains on a street covered with an archway of blooming jacaranda trees; their deep violet flowers shower down upon the car's windshield. *Oh, gorgeous springtime. Oh God, does that hurt!*

"Don't go over any more bumps!"

"That wasn't a bump," Joe tells me.

"It felt like a sinkhole. And why didn't they give me a graham cracker in the hospital so they could give me the pain pill there?" I ask him.

"We'll be home in five minutes."

"I don't want to wait. I need this pill now. Do you have any old crackers in the car? There's a water bottle right there on the floor."

"Hang on," Joe says. "Two minutes more." I lean back and fade out. The good thing is this: the cancer is out of me. That was the whole point of this operation. I'm on my way home. I'm done with needles and green operating rooms. I'm going right to my own soft bed.

But once we get into the house, I notice there's a nice soft couch even closer than my bed. I fall upon it. "Get me any sort of food, open a jar of apple sauce, get me water," I beg Joe. "I must swallow this pill."

In an hour, I'm much better. These pills—what is this magic? How could a small oblong white pill do something so mysterious and unbelievable as to erase a slash of pain? And not only that, it makes me feel peaceful and relaxed and utterly happy. I manage to get out of my clothes and put on a nightgown.

I get myself to the bathroom, and this is what I see in the mirror. It's not so bad, really. Two little bandages. One for the sentinel node, one for the place they removed the cancer. I still have my breast, it's still mine, and I'm still alive.

This isn't half as bad as I thought it would be.

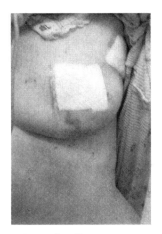

Day after first surgery

I float through the week, remembering very little of it. Sleeping, eating canned peaches, dozing, floating. Do my children call? I'm sure of it. Does Becky come to visit? No doubt, but I wave them all away, I'm fine, I'm drugged, I'm all fixed, I'm all better.

At the end of a week, I bravely remove the bandage. The scar is healing nicely. *Uh-oh, I see a little problem.* Where did my nipple go? It seems to have fallen into a deep depression and sunk out of sight. What now? Did my surgeon cut too far and fast? This was not supposed to happen. What now?

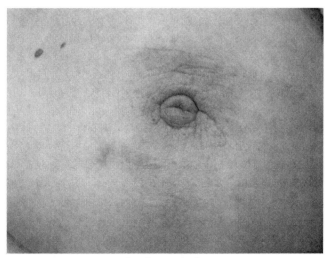

Sunken nipple

EIGHT
THE SECOND SURGERY
AND MORE SHOCKING NEWS

ODDS … WHAT DO THEY MEAN? IF seventy-five out of one hundred women don't need a second surgery "to get clean margins," how come I do? And if seventy-five out of one hundred women don't have the HER 2 neu (aggressive growth) factor, how come I do?

Joe says to look at it another way: to be born at all is against all odds—isn't it? To come into being is like winning a million lotteries at once. And yet, I counter Joe, my husband the history professor, about a passage I read in Sophocles' *Oedipus at Colonus*. I double check the quotation to make sure:

> Not to be born is best
> When all is reckoned in,
> But once a man has seen the light
> The next best thing, by far, is to go back,
> Back where he came from, as quickly as he can …

Joe and I have argued this before, in the matter of chickens. Consider all those chicken farms where millions of chickens are raised, just to be slaughtered. Joe's position is that it's worth it to the chickens to have a look around, worth basking in a beam of sunshine (if these chickens ever do), worth seeing trees and skies, even for a brief stay on earth.

But I'm not thinking chickens now, I'm thinking another surgery, scheduled exactly ten days from the first, which means in just a few days. The odds have foiled me. Again I will have to contend with the scrubbing-up packets for the showers, the re-slicing open of my breast, the bigger scoop my surgeon has to take this time to get "clean margins."

How much more do I want scooped out of my breast? And then again, what is this thing, this "aggressive growth factor"? There's always the internet to find out more:

> HER amplification or over-expression occurs in approximately 30% of breast cancers. It is strongly associated with increased disease recurrence and a worse prognosis.

Okay, right now I need real drugs, hard drugs, sleeping drugs, calming drugs, plus maybe a full tub of chocolate ice cream, or I may have to go into the backyard and cry, really cry, and make my dog-neighbor happy.

I call my surgeon. That is, I call her insofar as any medical patient can call her doctor these days—I send an email to her nurse with a request for her to call me.

An email is shortly returned. *At last, information!* But no, it is just the nurse acknowledging that she has received the email for the surgeon and that she will forward it to her.

"Worse prognosis"—the words burn in my breast, along with the healing, rough-edged tissue of my scar.

When the phone rings after dinner, I nearly rip it from the wall. But it's not my surgeon. It is my youngest daughter asking if she and her family can come and visit this weekend.

"No, of course not! I'm having surgery in a few days."

"Maybe the children can take your mind off it."

"What mind? I have no mind. Sweetheart, wait till afterward. I'll be sane then."

Suddenly I hear that call-waiting beep, that rude interruption of phone calls that gives a person the choice to dump his present caller in the hopes that the other caller will be a better deal. "I think it's my doctor. Talk to you later."

I hear the voice of my surgeon. She is calling me directly, possibly from her own home. She seems to want to apologize. "We can't really know if the margins are clean till the tumor is out, Merrill," she says. "We stain the sides of the tumor green, black, orange and blue—and if those dyes run to the very edge of the cut without an adequate margin, we have to go back in and get that clear margin. Then we know the cancer is out."

There is no arguing with her argument.

"But the HER 2 neu factor … that's terrible, isn't it?"

"Not really, not anymore," she replies. "Yes, if we didn't have this Herceptin drug it would be. In your case, you'd be what we call 'triple negative' since your tumor was not positive for either estrogen or progesterone treatment. But with Herceptin, which has been proven to target the over-expression of the HER 2 factor, we can get a very good result. What it does mean, though, is a year of treatment—an infusion every three weeks for a year."

A year sounds good to me in a strange way. She is implying I will still be alive in a year.

"But oh!" I tell her. "My nipple disappeared in the last surgery. Did you notice it sank way down into my breast?"

"I did," she said. "I'll take care of that. I'll put in a stitch or two, and it will be fine."

It will be fine, I think. *It will all be fine. I'm fine.* My daughter and my grandchildren will come to visit after the surgery. Life is fine. Life is worth having, without a doubt. I'm not a chicken. I will get to be in the sun for years after this is over.

"Do I really have to use those scrubbing-up packets?" I implore my surgeon. "I don't work in the mines; I don't work in a sewage plant. Two showers before surgery?"

"It's a wise thing to do." She tells me to have Joe pick the packets up at the hospital before my surgery. I want to beg, "Come on, can't we skip it this time?" But we can't.

There's another problem the day before surgery. It's April 13th. For some reason (I know the reason, the house is dirty) I have agreed to have my house cleaned by one of those teams of two women who drive up in a cute car with mops and brooms painted on the side. (We know the big company gets the big money and the working women get almost nothing.) Not only that, it is a Wednesday, the day my gardener comes to lop and chop. Not only that, but we have been late preparing our tax returns (with good reason) and someone from our tax man's office is coming to pick up our tax papers.

Is this not too much to face on the same day I have to take two showers to sterilize my germ-ridden body? To face having strangers in my house spraying toxic cleaners in my oven, toxic bleaches in my sinks and toilets? And the gardener, well, he is an old friend. He's been destroying my garden for at least ten years. He has only one general mode, which is to cast his eye on a bush, and if it's round and graceful, he cuts the top straight off. If it has a few stray branches (like my precious rosemary bush) he will pull the plant out by the roots, thinking it is a weed.

We do not keep him on for his aesthetic eye, but for his kindness, his wisdom, and his advice. When my daughter was in the process of adopting a child, he offered to pray for her; when our grandson arrived, he tipped his head and said, "You see, God has everything under control." Who could deny him that reasoning?

When tragedies that we both knew of occurred in the world, he said, "God thinks different than you and me. It's hard to be in the shoes of those suffering, but we can't try to understand these things." He was humble before the mysteries of life. It endeared him to me.

When, in the summertime, he spoke of his three daughters, as he often did, I asked him if he had any recent pictures of his family with him. He began to unbutton his shirt. He then pulled it off. On his enormously thick muscled arms he had tattoos of the faces of his daughters and his wife, and on his powerful back, a tattoo of Jesus.

Thus, outside, on this day before my second surgery, he and a younger man who helps him are chopping and grass-cutting and leaf-blowing: noise of the highest order. In the living room and kitchen and bathrooms, the team of cleaning ladies is vacuuming and spraying and scrubbing and flushing. Why is my bathtub so grimy? Why is the grout between the tiles full of mildew? Why do I have breast cancer? Why do I have to go back for another surgery?

Sitting in my office, in front of my computer, I begin to cry. Who can hear me anyway, with the blowers outside and the scrubbers inside? And then the doorbell rings and Joe opens it to give the tax man's helper our necessary papers. Our tax man is a Buddhist philosopher. In the months between tax seasons, he goes to meditative retreats at distant monasteries and tries to think of nothing, talk to no one, and eat brown rice. In his office, however, during tax season, he likes to talk to us in his office for a few hours and discuss the nature of life.

Joe comes to my door to ask me something about estimated tax forms for next year and finds me crying so hard the keys on my computer are glowing with teardrops.

What can a husband do at such a time? My office is such a tangle of papers, so many mountains of books are piled on every surface, so many fortune-cookie fortunes and paperclips are flung around the room. The big wooden devil-chaser my father gave me from his antique store (to keep me safe) blocks the way. Joe cannot even get close to me. I cry and he watches me. I can see the puzzlement on his face. I can see his pain and bafflement. He can't possibly understand what someone who has cancer is going through that causes her to cry her eyes out.

NINE
A PERKY NIPPLE AND A LONG ROAD AHEAD

FLOWERS ARRIVE FROM FRIENDS.

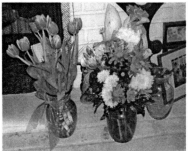

Flowers from friends

Not only that, I discover that my nipple has cleverly risen to the surface under the guidance of my surgeon's precise stitch. I am quite heartened by this.

I am done with surgery, done with scrubbing up showers, done with scalpels and being asked if I am a ten or less. Now I get to heal and think of other things. Think of a visit with my youngest daughter and her family.

But when my daughter and her family arrive, I am a limp and floppy thing. Do I want to walk to the park with them? (It's only one block away, right next to the Pioneer Cemetery.) I demur.

I seem to want to stay in bed. I don't feel like crying, nor do

I feel like watching my adorable granddaughter and fearless grandson climb on the playground climbing wall or swing on the playground swings. Nor does television interest me, or reading, or anything but resting and perhaps sleeping.

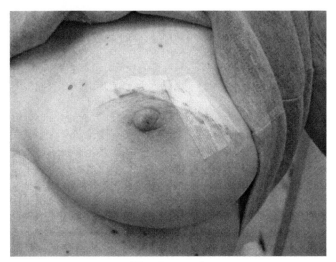

Nipple cured

My granddaughter, who is three, looks exactly like my daughter (her mother) looked at three, and I have fantasies of being a young mother again, of feeling those delicious little arms being raised up to me, of holding that solid little weight in my lap so the pages of a book can be turned by both of us. They tease each other, mother and daughter, about the baby blanket, which each one claims is hers. "I need it!" says my daughter. "I need it!" says my granddaughter. She laughs with mad abandon. The game goes on, getting louder.

"No, I need it!"

"No, I need it!"

But I need quiet. Where, in a house where houseguests are staying, is there quiet?

My grandson and his father are trying to catch butterflies and lizards in the backyard. All my margarine containers have been commandeered for use as little prisons for a "cabbage," for a "fritillary," for one of undisclosed stripes. The rule is the creatures must all be freed within a half hour. No lizards are captured—they're simply too fast.

Food—there's an issue, and it comes up every few hours. I defer to my kids—they'll figure it out, pick up a roasted chicken, or my son-in-law will whip up something with pasta and sauce. He's a great cook. It's odd—I used to own my kitchen, but now there's a "free for all" in there and I don't care. I'm not in charge. I'm not the hostess anymore, more like a guest.

Not that I really want to eat. Not that I really want to do "Knock, Knock" jokes with my grandson. I have entered a new reality where something enormous awaits me.

And I know what it is. It's the appointment with the oncologist, with the cancer doctor. She has a name, I swear it, that seems to me to sound like Dr. Crap. She's the next step in the series of rungs I must climb. Surgeon, oncologist, radiologist, then cardiologist. Chemo and radiation can damage a woman's heart. Tests must be done at intervals to see how the heart is faring. Cancer is dangerous, but a stopped heart is the end of the line. We've got to have a balance sheet made up for us by my doctors. We've got to consider these calculations next week after the children leave.

I hide in my bed. Though the door is closed, my granddaughter pushes it open. She's holding her blankie. She throws it, a ragged blue thing, on my bed. Then she grabs it back.

"I need it!" she says. And she waits.

"I need it!" I say, joining her game, grabbing and pulling on her blanket, and she laughs a child's laughter that tinkles with golden bells.

"Can Grandma give you a kiss?" I ask her. She happily approaches the bed and presents her cheek to me. I kiss her. *God, how much I love her and life and all my children and their children and my husband and laughter and beauty.* How could one contemplate the end of it all? It cannot be done. Instead, lists must be made, statistics must be considered, survival rates must be laid on the line. All this to ask the oncologist. But really, there is just one question on the list. *I have cancer. Will I live?*

TEN
THE WRONG DOCTOR FOR ME

T HIS IS THE DAY I AM to meet—so far as I understand it—
the captain of my ship. She will guide my passage through
the rocky byways of cancer treatment and lead me to safety on
the other side. I am waxing poetic, feeling on the brink of some
momentous relationship. My life will be in this woman's hands, as
it already has been in my surgeon's. Joe and I bring our trusty old
cassette recorder, and in it is a new tape. I set the recorder on the
regulation cabinet that is in every examining room, next to the
computer on a stand that is now a requirement as well.

When Dr. Carp finally arrives in the room, she heads straight
for the computer. She neither looks at us nor shakes our hands.
After a period of typing ensues, I say, quite tentatively, "I'm
Merrill."

"I know," she says.

"I have some questions to ask you."

"I'm not ready," she says.

Joe and I look at each other, and then at Dr. Carp. She is about
sixty, I would guess, with bleached yellow hair flying loose down
her back. She is sitting on a stool that is at computer-keyboard
height, and Joe and I are in green plastic chairs. After ten minutes
pass, I say, "Would it be all right if I tape what you tell me?"

"I prefer not," she says.

It's a new world, this doctor-at-her-computer, her eyes on the screen rather than on me, her fingers on the keyboard rather than on me. Writing the history of the patient takes place *during* the visit, not after, and the old-fashioned "Get dressed and come into my office" experience has vanished with the advent of technology. What's odd is that the doctor is doing her work on my time, not on hers. I have to sit by and wait while she does her homework, or so it seems.

There is not much to do while she types. What's the scenery in here? On the wall shelf, blue latex gloves are on display in small, medium, and large sizes. Once in the past, while awaiting a doctor, I dragged a few gloves out of the box and stuffed them in my purse. I had an idea what I wanted them for. For example, if I dropped my hairbrush in the toilet, I could put on a pair of those blue gloves in order to retrieve it. If I needed to stick my fingers in a drain, mud hole, or any other unpleasant place, I could imagine needing those gloves. The yellow rubber gloves I have for cleaning up the kitchen would not serve as well.

Now I realize that stealing those gloves may be why I have cancer. There may be many reasons I have cancer, but how can I ever know which one put me over the line? Stealing gloves? Eating an excess of nitrite-treated kosher hot dogs? Living at a time when cigarette smoke choked us in every public place?

Decades earlier, I had been an active member of GASP—*Group Against Smoking Pollution*. I carried a little battery-run fan in my purse. At restaurants, when waves of cigarette smoke came my way, I would turn on the fan and send the smoke back toward the smoker. One day, as I drove on the freeway with a GASP bumper sticker on my car, someone honked at me. I looked to my right and saw a man with his head sticking out the driver's window. He had a cigarette hanging out of his mouth, two hanging out of his nostrils, and two sticking out of his ears. His message to me was clear.

Still, it took forever for the world to take notice that smoke was killing us.

So, did smoke give me cancer? Did lox? Maybe driving behind

diesel trucks did. How could anyone drive behind such a vehicle, inhaling as it belched forth clouds of black poison, and not get sick?

Dr. Carp is still typing. I clear my throat. "I have so many questions to ask you," I say.

"I'm not ready," she replies, typing. Typing slowly, in fact. Personally, I am a speedy and enthusiastic typist. I won the typing medal when I graduated from high school. The award is in my jewel box: a gold pin in the shape of a typewriter with the number "60" on it. Typing sixty words a minute in high school was medal-worthy.

Of course, I thought I should have been awarded the English medal, but being recognized for typing made me happy enough. I love typewriters and cherish all of them I have ever owned. In my collection now are the Smith Corona I took to college; the Remington; the Underwood; the little light Olivetti I carried with me to shady parks where I could type on a picnic table.

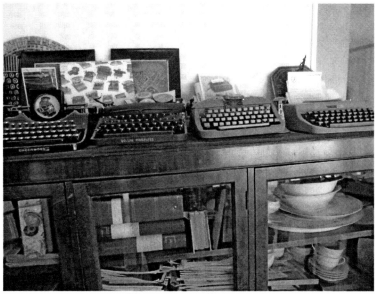
Typewriter collection

Best of all my typewriters was my beloved electric typewriter with which I was blessed. Many years ago Joe and I passed an IBM typewriter store. I looked longingly at the IBM *Selectric* on display, a magical machine that had abandoned the carriage return and instead featured a spinning silver ball that danced back and forth across the page.

The salesman could see I was smitten. "Let me lend you one for just a week, with no obligation," he offered. "I'll deliver it and set it up for you. Then, at the end of a week I'll come and get it. No obligation of any sort."

I agreed. I gave him my address and I made a pact with myself. If I could write a short story on it and sell it, I would buy a *Selectric*.

The salesman delivered the machine to me. I was awed by its bright blue color. He left me a selection of spinning balls, each with a different font. I sat down and within a few days, I wrote a short story. A month later, when I learned from *Redbook* that they wanted to buy it, I called the salesman. "Deliver a *Selectric* to me, please. I'd like one in light brown."

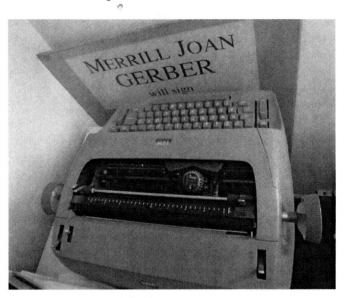

Selectric typewriter

Finally, Dr. Carp stops typing. She stands and leaves the room without a word.

"Something's wrong here," I say to Joe. I look out the window. Down below is a pond that surrounds the medical center and the hospital. A single duck glides on the water. It seems to be there as a symbol of health and hope.

Dr. Carp returns to the examining room carrying a sheaf of papers. She pulls up her stool next to my chair and shakes the papers in my direction. "I've determined that you will need a cocktail of three chemo drugs—Taxol, Carboplatin, and Herceptin." She hands me three sets of papers, each set stapled together. Then, on the examining table, she lays a sheet of paper labeled with my name, my age, my tumor size (1.1-2.0 centimeters), my estrogen receptor status: (Negative), my Histological Grade (3) and my nodes involved (0).

She taps the sheet of paper. It is titled: "Shared Decision Making Regarding Breast Cancer."

"Please read this."

Joe and I look at the shaded chart she displays for us. It seems to offer my statistics for survival.

Decision: No additional therapy
47 out of 100 women are alive and without cancer in ten years.
27 out of 100 women relapse.
26 out of 100 women die of other causes.
Decision: Hormonal Therapy
Less than 1 out of 100 women are alive and without cancer because of therapy.

Decision: Chemotherapy—Third Generation Regimen
10 out of 100 women are alive and without cancer because of therapy.
Decision: Combined therapy
10 out of 100 women are alive and without cancer because of therapy.

I look at Joe and he looks at me. What is this all about? I don't understand a word of it.

"If I take all these chemo drugs," I ask Dr. Carp, "what would my life expectancy be?"

"I don't discuss mortality," she says.

"You don't?"

"Please read the side effects of these drugs now. I need to know that you understand what you may experience."

I look at the information about Carboplatin:

> Warning: This medicine is very strong. It can prevent your bone marrow from making cells that your body needs. You will be closely monitored by healthcare provider. Tell provider right away about any fever, sore throat, signs of infection, bleeding, shortness of breath. Dangerous allergic reactions can occur. Carboplatin injures cancer cells causing their death. Tell your provider if you feel very tired.

"I feel tired right now," I say. Dr. Carp stares at me. Her expression does not waver. She nods toward the paper, indicating that I must read further. Joe and I read together:

> Reasons to call healthcare provider immediately:
> Severe nausea
> Severe vomiting
> Severe diarrhea
> Severe cough
> Unusual bruising or bleeding
> Dark urine or yellow skin
> Not able to eat
> No improvement in condition or feeling worse
>
> What are some common side effects:
> Nausea
> Skin irritation
> Hair loss
> Anemia, low white blood cell count and low platelet count

"You will also want to read the side effects of the other drugs," Dr. Carp says, "and then you might have some questions for me."

I glance at the other pages for Herceptin (also called Trastuzumab) and for Taxol (Docetaxel). They have their own warnings and alarms about side effects:

> Muscle pain, Mouth ulcers, Runny nose, Belly pain, Feeling dizzy, Headache, Not hungry, Chest pain, Fast heartbeat, Severe dizziness or passing out, Significant weight gain, Chills, Severe mouth sores, Painful urination, Wound that will not heal, Swelling of face, lips, tongue or throat.

"My God," I say to Dr. Carp.

"Well," she says, crossing her arms across her chest, "*It's not candy.*"

WE STOP FOR GAS ON THE way home. "I won't have her as my doctor," I tell Joe. I put some bills in the cash slot next to the pump.

"Of course not."

"So what do I do next?"

Joe is watching the numbers fly by on the gas pump display. A boy of about sixteen approaches us, carrying a box.

"Would you like to buy some candy to help the blind?"

"I have *cancer*," I say to him. "I'm not buying candy!"

A look of shock crosses his face. When I glance at Joe, he too seems shocked.

"Do you really have cancer?" the boy asks. "Are you going to live?"

"I don't know yet."

"What kind is it?"

"Breast." The word seems to shock him even more.

"I hope you live. I'll pray for you."

"That's nice of you." I get into the car. I think he should give me a free box of candy. I think perhaps I should give him five dollars.

He is so young, and I made him think he had looked into the face of death.

Candy, I think. Oh indeed, chemo is *not* candy.

ELEVEN
THE CANCER SUPPORT COMMUNITY

W HAT OUR FACILITATOR SAYS TO ME in my support group
when I tell the story about my comment to the boy selling
candy is: "That's called playing the cancer card."

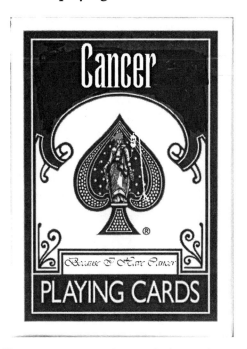

"Cancer card" image courtesy of Peg Schulte, author and journalist,
whose own book, *A Guide to playing the Cancer Card*, is in progress

"But why did I do it?" I ask.

"Many people do it," she says. "It's a way of getting out of an obligation, or a way of not having to stand in line, or even to avoid getting a traffic ticket. It's a way of getting some use out of cancer, which sucks, as we all know."

Once again, in the same way I can't say for sure how I found the lump in my breast, I don't recall how I found the Cancer Support Community. A friend who had been there might have recommended it to me. A nurse in the Oncology Department might have suggested I go there. A little messenger might have taken my hand and led me to their door.

In any case, after meeting Dr. Carp, I feel desperately in need of support. I call the Cancer Support Community, and they urge us to come. After a brief interview with a man who has survived several serious cancers, we are assigned to our groups—I to a cancer patient group and Joe to a caregivers group.

We are to meet once a week, in the evening, in a suite of rooms, all of them having a homey feeling. A grand piano is present in what seems like a living room. On it, some pink "Cancer Survivor" bracelets sit in a small bowl. Soft chairs and two couches are arranged around a coffee table displaying issues of free magazines named *Cure* and *Cancer Guide*. In the hallway are brochures about weekly programs: guided meditation, yoga for sleep, knitting nirvana, qi gong, tai chi, dynamic strength training, and watercolor painting—and some special programs as well, on medical marijuana, photography, modern dance, and hospice care. Lectures are coming up on complementary and natural therapies, eating a plant-based diet, and drinking non-acidic water. One is called "Chemo Brain, What Is it?" and "The Boogie Man in the Closet: Facing Death." Another announces: "Look Good, Feel Better!"

"Lots to do here," I say to Joe.

He looks dubious. He is not a man to discuss his feelings openly, much less with a group of strangers. He is just learning to face his fears and concerns, one on one, with me. He hasn't yet, technically, become my caregiver (unless you count all the years of our marriage and maybe, in that context, it is the other way around).

But we split up, he going to his group and I going to the one that will become my home once a week for the indefinite future. There is a pattern to these meetings: our facilitator has each person already in the group introduce himself/herself to the new member (me) by explaining the nature of his/her disease and how long he/she has been in treatment. Then it is my turn. At this point, I am an early player in the game. Only a biopsy and two surgeries. And Dr. Carp. I tell them the story.

"It's not candy!" they repeat in astonishment, one by one. My group (already it feels like "my group") tells me what I have to do: get a new oncologist.

Well, of course. A great weight lifts from me. Cancer sucks, they assure me, and there are all kinds of things I will have to face along the way. The rule is "Be proactive." Make noise, make waves, make trouble, make war. This is a life and death battle, right? Get armed in every way. And the first way to arm yourself is to get a doctor who cares if you live or die.

Our meeting room has an incredible vibration of concern in it. Our leader is a loving woman whose breasts were removed not so long ago. She is a guarantee that one can survive such massacres. We are already like relatives, family, or better—dear old friends. I have just heard descriptions of their tremendous troubles: pancreatic cancer, ovarian cancer, naso-pharyngeal cancer, brain cancer, thyroid cancer, colon cancer, anal cancer. There are two women with breast cancer, like me. One, who is eighty-three, is a powerhouse of humor and vitality. Her cancer had been cured, and then a new, unrelated one, came back six years later.

Several of the women wear scarves around their heads. One, it is clear, is wearing a wig—a purple wig, in fact. There is a sense of bonding I've never felt in any other group, and it warms the room. There are soft fleecy blankets around the room, as well, for those needing a sense of protection or for those having the side effects of chills. At the meeting's end, after I am inducted into the club where cancer is "the new reality," our group gathers in a circle and wraps their arms around one another. And, standing there on a little table, in the center of our circle, is a lovely sculpture of embracing figures in a circle, their arms wrapped around one another.

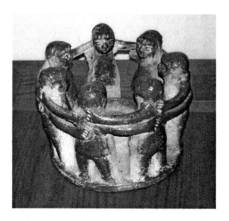

Loving circle cancer support community

TWELVE
SAINT BELINDA OF THE BATTERIES

BREASTS, OF COURSE, ARE NOT THE only important essence in this machine of a body we live our lives in. Years ago, on a walk around the block with Joe, I felt extremely short of breath. I had to sit down on the curb. I could hardly get myself home.

Though I felt better the next morning, I made an appointment with my cardiologist, and two days later I drove myself to his office. He asked his nurse to do an EKG. When he read it, he said (quietly, and seriously) that it looked as if I might have had a heart attack. We had to see what was going on. He made a phone call and arranged for me to have an angiogram the next day.

When I left his office, I was trembling. I passed a room where a cardiology tech was doing something—she took one look at me and came out into the hall.

"Honey, what's wrong?"

"My cardiologist thinks I may have had a heart attack," I told her.

She put her arms around me and led me into the room. "Please," she said, "just sit right here for a minute." She was a stunningly beautiful black woman with eyes that shone liquid with compassion.

"You just rest and get your breath back."

She seemed to be working on something—she was holding a

little device, black and rectangular. From it she took four little batteries, put them on the counter, and then, taking four batteries from another box, inserted them into the device.

"What a waste," she explained to me. "These are for Holter monitors. A patient wears them for twenty-four hours to monitor their heart rhythm. These batteries can be used only once and then have to be thrown out. They're almost brand new, but the rule is that we have to put in new batteries for each new patient."

I shrugged. Who cared about batteries? "I have to have an angiogram tomorrow," I told her. "Dr. Cotter ordered it."

She studied my face. "Listen," she said, "your doctor is the best. Whatever he's going to do for you, you'll be just fine. In fact, you're fine right now. Look at you, your color is good, you can walk, you can talk. Would you like some free batteries?"

"Would I?"

They're very useful. They're triple A's, the kind you can use in lots of things—the TV remote or a little flashlight or a radio."

"Don't you need them?"

"No. I have to throw them away." She began packing some up, in groups of four, in the little empty boxes that the new ones had come in. I read her name tag under her ID photo that hung around her neck: Belinda Blue.

"Here, open your purse." She dropped a bunch of little battery boxes in my purse. She hugged me again. "Don't you worry, sweetheart, you'll be just fine."

Joe took me for the angiogram the next morning—I hadn't had a heart attack. Something else had caused the strange EKG reading, but it wasn't going to kill me. When in two weeks, I returned for a follow-up appointment, I asked to speak to Belinda. They called her out to the waiting room for me.

"I just want to tell you, you were right. I'm fine and I didn't have a heart attack."

Belinda hugged me. I could feel the comfort of her strong body. I just wanted to lean against her for a few minutes. "Honey, I'll give you some more batteries. You can never have too many," she whispered in my ear. "Just come with me."

* * *

AFTER MY ENCOUNTER WITH THE TERRIBLE Dr. Carp, I call my cardiologist.

"I can't have her for my oncologist," I tell him. "She's poison. Do you know of another oncologist who might be right for me?"

"My mother has a great one," he tells me. "Right here in this building."

"Your mother has cancer?"

"Yes, she's doing very well," he says.

"Can you tell me who her doctor is?"

"We all call her Dr. B. You'll find she's terrific."

I feel a rush of joy. If she is caring for my cardiologist's mother, how can she be wrong for me?

THIRTEEN
THE BLESSED DOCTOR B

THIS IS MY FIRST GLIMPSE OF Dr. B. On the day of my initial
appointment with her, I leave the waiting room and walk
down the hall in the Oncology Department, looking for the
restroom.

I pass an open office door. Inside is a woman sitting at her
desk, eating lunch. Her feet are in flip-flops. Holding a can of soda
in her hand, she glances up at me. She smiles and tips her drink.
I smile back. Something happy has happened in me, something
hopeful. Another dear stranger in this HMO—a place designed
to take care of people, to take care of me.

Joe and I are waiting in an examining room when there's a
knock at the door. The woman in flip-flops comes in. Her face is
as bright as the sun.

Somehow, I extend my arms toward her and she comes and
hugs me. She wears her white doctor's coat over a shirt and pair of
short slacks—pedal pushers we called them in my youth. When
she lets go of me, she shakes Joe's hand.

"Well, here we are." She doesn't type a word on the computer
in the room. She sits and talks to us for an hour. She explains all
the forthcoming treatments I'll be offered, the best ones for my
type of cancer. She refers to some pages printed out beforehand
and points out to me the kinds of chemo I will be getting. We will

start at weekly intervals, once a week for six weeks, and then once every three weeks for a year. Yes, there are difficult side effects, but there are medications to counter all of them—anti-nausea drugs for nausea, opioids for pain, injections to help red-blood cells regenerate, and sleeping pills for the times I can't sleep. A team of special oncology pharmacists will be on call to give advice about dosages of my medications or for simple reassurance that those I'm taking can be combined with others.

"These treatments are designed to kill the fast-growing cells in your body. They are aimed primarily at the cancer cells, but some other cells will of course be affected, including your hair cells." I'll lose my hair in about two weeks. My digestive tract will be affected, and food might taste funny for a while. If ever, during treatment, I get a fever above 100.5, I am to go to the Emergency Room. "Just say you have a fever and you're on chemo. They'll know what to do."

The first chemo treatment, which she schedules for May 11th, will be administered very slowly; it will take about six hours. I will be given meds to make me a bit sleepy, and that will counter any allergic reactions to the chemo drugs—the Taxol, the Carboplatin, and the Herceptin. After my treatment, I should eat things that appeal to me. Chocolate energy drinks are good; protein is important. She will prescribe a magic mouth rinse that will numb any blisters I might get in my mouth. It seems she has thought of everything and has told me everything she wants me to think about.

"And a year from now," she says, "you'll wonder why you were so frightened today." She gives me her sunny smile. "Any questions?"

"I love your face," I say. "Would you mind if we took a picture together?"

I get my camera out of my purse and hand it to Joe. I didn't bring my tape recorder but there has been no need. The picture of Dr. B is all I wanted.

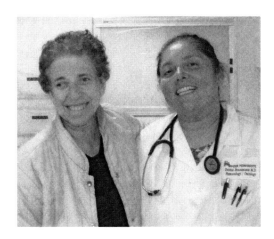

Merrill and Dr. B

FOURTEEN
FIRST DAY IN CHEMO CHAIR

THIS OF COURSE IS THE MOMENTOUS moment: poison will be pumped into my veins and will disseminate, like an army of fierce soldiers carrying bayonets, to stab, one by one, the sly and canny cancer cells hiding wherever my bloodstream may have carried them. The battle cry is everywhere. Pick any obituary column and you will read: "Died after a long battle with cancer." Or more terrifying, "Died after a brief battle with cancer."

I am not dressed for battle—comfortable clothes, my instruction sheet says. "Prepare for a six-hour infusion the first day. Wear clothing that allows access to your arm. Wear no jewelry."

But wait: I am already wearing the assigned jewelry—the pink rubbery bracelet advised for all breast cancer patients that says, "No needles, no blood pressure."

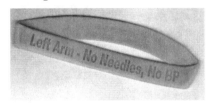

Left Arm, No needles, No BP

My left arm, on the side of my left breast, is now off-limits for life. Lymphedema is the danger. Once lymph nodes are removed to check for cancer, the lymph system is permanently disturbed—lymph can ooze anywhere once its normal channels are disturbed. Two women in my cancer support group wear tight elastic bandages on their upper arms, but these women had many lymph nodes removed, as many as twenty-two. In one case, cancer was found in all of them.

I had only the one sentinel node removed; I am less at risk. But still, left arm, no needles, no blood pressure. A small inconvenience, of course, at this point, but other things will happen to my body—I am just at the start of the obstacle course. There's no knowing what will happen.

Joe and I try to find the infusion room. We know it's at a far corner on the third floor of the hospital building. It's actually hard to get there, a long walk from the parking structure to the building, a long circle around the lobby—where a player-piano, roped off, plays monotonal tunes from the old days—a long walk down a hallway past the lab, past the pharmacy, past the Orthopedic Department—inside we see young kids waiting with casts on their arms and legs—and to some elevators opposite the Emergency Room.

I'm tired already, and I haven't even started chemo. Joe is carrying my supplies: my little bag of crackers and juice, my book to read, my fuzzy pink fleece blanket. This last is a present from a friend. When she learned I had cancer, she delivered to my door a small package of caps and hats and the special blanket that her mother used during her chemo: "I wanted her to have something soft and something from home so she would feel safe." However, her mother died of her breast cancer, after her "long battle."

As soon as I find my assigned chair in the chemo room, a nurse arrives with a pillow for my head and two heated cotton blankets, which she arranges tenderly over my body. She adjusts the chair I am in and the chair reclines, the footrest pops up. Already I feel better: warmer and more relaxed. I tell Joe to put the pink fleece blanket back in my carry bag. I don't want to use it.

A plastic bracelet is affixed to my arm. An army of nurses, men and women, are attending to patients. One is assigned to me. Her name is Cristina. Already I love her, I can tell by her touch on my arm that she is gentle, efficient. She admires my red hat and my red sweater—the color of blood, I think. I want my blood to be full of bravery today, to accept the killer drugs that will join up with my red and white blood cells and travel with them to wipe out every last enemy cell. Just this one time, I've left my four-leaf clover necklace at home.

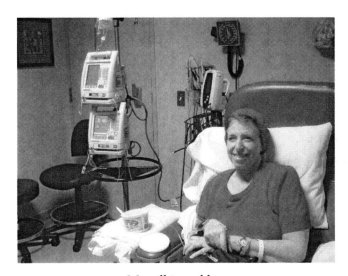

Merrill in red hat

There is a protocol here: I have already had my blood pressure and temperature taken. Cristina examines my plastic bracelet. I examine it, too.

She then calls over another nurse to verify what is on it. The nurse reads aloud my name, my birth date, my age, today's date, my sex, my medical record number. Then Cristina takes my right arm, rests it on a small table, and does what she has to do: she brings over her equipment—needles, tape, sterile wipes—finds an available vein, cleans the skin with a sterile wipe, and gives me a gentle warning: "A little sharp stick now." I hold Joe's hand with my left hand and feel the needle go in. "Take a deep breath," Cristina says. She wiggles the needle slightly. "We're in," she says, with a note of triumph. She tapes the needle in place, covers it with a clear plastic strip to secure it, and goes to order my IV medicine.

Then I am given my meds by mouth, Benadryl and some cortisone pills. After this, we will wait about a half hour. The pharmacy has to make up the infusion combination. It can't be done till the needle is in place.

While we wait, we look around. Right next to me is an older woman, a woman about my age. We are all older women, aren't we? She smiles at me from her chair. "I'm Maria," she says.

"I'm Merrill. Nice to meet you," I reply. Her medicine is already being administered. She seems quite cheerful about it. In fact, all the patients in this infusion room seem cheerful. One or two are dozing. Others have a friend or a relative with them and are talking quite happily. No one looks sick. No one looks as if she is dying. One woman is doing embroidery. Another is reading.

Maria suddenly hands me something. "What is it?"

"Take this and eat it," she says. "You are going to need a lot of strength. You'll be here a while the first time."

I discover I'm holding a margarine container. In it is pink yogurt and a plastic spoon. I don't feel like eating, but I open it and take a few spoonfuls.

"Some days," she says, "you won't be able to eat anything. So when you can, you eat!" I spoon more strawberry yogurt into my mouth. "Your sense of taste will change," she warns me, "so don't be surprised if everything tastes like a metal doorknob."

"What is your illness?" I ask her. "I'm here for breast cancer."

"Lung cancer," she says. "Because for twenty years I worked in Nicaragua rolling cigars. I'm an expert at it. I made the best cigars in the world."

"Did you smoke them?"

"No, but I was around them all the time and around people smoking them. I even tasted the leaves. We have a cigar store now, my husband and I. Right here in El Monte."

Maria fishes in her purse and hands me a business card. I glance at it and hand it to Joe. "Thanks very much," I say. Joe puts it in his shirt pocket.

Now my medicine has arrived. Nurse Cristina shows me the first bag of it, a clear liquid, as she hangs it on a silver hook attached to some machinery. She calls over another nurse and the nurse scans some identifying numbers on it with a wand. It is hung next to a bag of saline solution that Cristina says I will also be getting, along with my medication. She pushes a button. A timer begins to tick.

There we go. Drip by drip, my chemo drug slides down the clear thin tube and into my bloodstream. We've begun the battle to the death.

FIFTEEN
"AM I DEAD YET?"
MY BEST FRIEND DIES OF CANCER

I AM NOT THE FIRST OF MY generation facing cancer. At Miami Beach High School, Martha and I were best friends, the kind who were constantly talking on the phone and in school and eating meals with each other, although I ate at her home more often. Her mother was a loving cook and always had delicious and special foods at their house. Martha's parents had a business in Cuba and were often away. Martha and her beautiful little sister, Betsy, had a good amount of freedom. I remember how we played *The Student Prince* album over and over. We loved to hear Mario Lanza sing those romantic songs and we dreamed of our own romances.

Martha had a car, a blue and white Chevrolet. She drove us to school and saved me from taking the school bus. We double-dated—I with Joe, whom I adored, and Martha with one or another of the nice young men from Miami Beach High School. A date in those days for us consisted of our having hot fudge sundaes at some diner and then choosing a fancy hotel on the Miami Beach. We'd go through the lobby and out the back to the pool area, where there were cabanas and beach chairs. The four of us would sit quietly, staring at the moon dancing over the ocean, and we dreamed whatever dreams we had then of our futures, which would be wonderful and full of love. Now and then some kissing might ensue, but it was virtuous and sweet.

After graduation, Martha went away to college in Wisconsin and I to the University of Florida. We wrote to each other, long letters full of confidences. Somehow life parted us and then brought us together again. Somehow she moved to California, and so did I. The first time I visited her in Los Angeles, each of us had a baby girl. When I arrived at Martha's house, she saw me coming up the steps with my daughter Becky in my arms and she cried out, "Look what you have!"

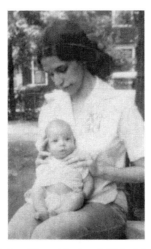

Merrill and baby, MJG shirt

And I looked at beautiful baby Michelle in her arms and replied, "And look what you have!" It was a moment of such bliss.

Having babies meant we had fallen in love, we had married, we'd had sex. The things had come to pass that we worried in high school might never come to pass. I married Joe, the boy we had double-dated with. Now, more than fifty years later, almost too many years to count, he was still the boy I adored. Martha and I could be apart even for a year or two, and then, when we met, we simply resumed our old intimacy without a missed beat. We simply loved each other, always and forever.

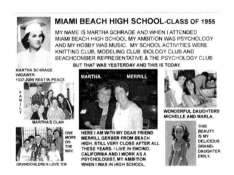

Martha high school page

We never dreamed life could deal us such a bitter blow as was dealt too early to her. She was still young, as young as I was. We were still teenage girls. Where did her cancer come from? And why did it devour her so fast?

"My life is upside down," she wrote to me in an email. "I think I'm done for."

I called her at once, and she was so tired she could hardly speak to me on the phone. A day later she was in the ICU, dying. Her sister told me that in the hospital she kept asking, "Am I dead yet? Why is it taking so long?" I knew that last phrase; she had said it to me many times in high school: "Why don't I have a boyfriend yet? Why is it taking so long?" And later she said, "Why am I not pregnant yet? Why is it taking so long?"

My sweet darling Martha was buried in the Jewish cemetery where my mother and father are buried.

As Mario Lanza used to sing, "Beloved, with all my heart I love you …"

That's how I feel about Martha.

SIXTEEN
CHEMO—NOTHING TO IT

L OOK AT ME, I'VE HAD CHEMO and I'm fit as a fiddle. The very
next day I go with Joe to a dermatology appointment so he
can have some black moles on his body examined. The doctor
can't be sure it isn't melanoma. She excises both moles.

I tell her I had my first chemo yesterday—*we can't both have
cancer* is my subtext. Please, not the two of us at once. Joe *has* to
be the caregiver. I'm not up for it right now.

We go to lunch at our favorite Mexican restaurant—time may
be shorter than money, we reason, so let's start living high and
spending our fortune. I gaze with appreciation upon the Mexican
decorations, the hanging wooden parrots, the ads for Mexican
beer, the paintings on the walls. My gaze lingers on one painting
of two old folks looking into each other's eyes.

However, if I look closely, I can see hidden in the face of the
old man the young and handsome man. His eyebrow is the curve
of his sombrero, and the angle of his nose is transformed into his
arm playing on a guitar a love song to his lovely lady. And look
there: where the old woman's eye should be, there is the young girl
holding up her hat and listening to his love song.

I look at Joe, my beloved since the beginning of time, and see
in his face the boy of my passion all these years. We are so old.

We are coming to the end of our journey; we—one or the other of us—will be left alone. Who will die first?

Joe, however, is a guy and has a certain guy-like approach. Why talk about it now? Why waste a perfectly nice time—dinner, walk, snuggle, car ride—by pre-living our deaths? It makes no sense.

But what if I'm left alone in my house, which I will suddenly hate—hate every room, every piece of furniture, every picture on the wall, every sock in every drawer. On the other hand, what if he is left alone and eats nothing but canned soup for every meal the rest of his life? He will die of salt poisoning, at the very least. On the other hand, what if he goes online to Match.com or JDate and finds a twenty-five-year-old girlfriend? What if she finds all my old earrings not to her taste and tosses them into the recycle bin? Or what if she likes them and begins wearing them? My pair of tiny hummingbird earrings? Or the earrings we bought in Florence, Italy, that look like buttons that belong on a brocade couch? But she'll be young and of course have pierced ears. Many piercings per ear, in fact, whereas my earrings are all clip-ons.

I could cry, just thinking of her—whoever she might be, though the one I imagine will of course be young and beautiful—lying on my side of the bed. Yet, to be fair and generous, I should wish for my husband a happy life after I'm dead. He should wish the same for me. But no, I will not start dating again at my age. I will not worry about my hairstyle. In fact, the very truth is that in a couple of weeks I will have no hair. Maybe no eyebrows, as well. I will probably have peripheral neuropathy, one of the side effects of chemo, and I will have no feeling in my peripheral parts. I will have numb lips that won't be much good for kissing. I already have a scarred breast I don't want any stranger fooling around with, and whoever I might be dating after Joe dies can just as well leave the other side alone, too.

The truth is I don't want to die. I don't want Joe to die. I don't, in fact, want anyone I love to die, or even anyone now alive on earth to die, though I wouldn't miss the dog neighbor if she never showed up again.

The waiter brings our food: chili relleno, rice and beans for me, and mojarra for Joe, an entire fried fish laid out on the plate with a cooked white eye looking up at him. I don't know how two people with such divergent tastes could have lived together for so many years. I would never tackle a whole dead fish and have to pick among the scales and bones (and little teeth!) for my dinner. Once, when I was a child, my grandmother got a fishbone stuck in her throat. They had to rush her to the doctor's house. (He lived two houses away, which was the way of life in Brooklyn in those days.) He got her to eat some soft white bread, and it pushed the bone down. The mushy bread coated the bone so it wouldn't stick in her insides, and she was just fine. But still, I avoid fishbones as if my life depended upon it.

What *does* my life depend upon? As of this week, Carboplatin, Taxol and Herceptin. This cancer cocktail is already coursing through my bloodstream like a fierce school of little fish-eyes, all of them wide open, seeking the enemy.

My chile relleno is too spicy tonight; I think the chef used a hotter pepper than usual. Something must be making my eyes tear; I don't know what it is. In fact, I'm not even hungry. Joe is happily poking among the bones of his dead fish and I am looking at that picture on the wall of the old man and the old woman who used to be young lovers.

I want to go home and go to bed. I am no longer feeling fit as a fiddle. In fact, I feel confused. There's a condition I've read about called "chemo-brain." I don't know how fast it comes on, but I think it's here right now and I think I have already fallen victim to it.

SEVENTEEN
THIS IS HOW BAD IT IS

WITHOUT MY MEMORY—CHEMO BRAIN HAS ALREADY destroyed my memory—I can't remember what happened after the first chemo infusion. Nothing happens at first—that much I do remember. During the first week, the dermatologist who looked at Joe's black moles calls us up—she calls me personally, she doesn't even ask to talk to Joe—to assure me that he doesn't have melanoma. "He's fine, it's nothing, don't worry. I hope you get through your treatment and get well."

How often does a doctor call you up to give you happy news? What does she secretly know about my treatment she isn't telling me? She wants to take away some percentage of my fear and worry. But I'm afraid and I don't worry. I'm suddenly too sick.

Later, when I try to remember what happened, I draw a smoky blank. That's what I see in my mind—darkness and a swirling feeling of desperation. This is what is written in my medical record:

> Seven days after patient's first chemo treatment she was having diarrhea and mouth sores. She was unable to eat. Her white blood count was low. Her blood pressure was 73/37, pulse 95. She had abnormal liver function test results. She had a fever. She had a urinary tract infection.

She received IV hydration and a shot of neupogen to elevate white blood cell count. She was given "miracle mouthwash" for her mouth sores. She was instructed to return the next day to be rechecked.

When patient returned the next day she was admitted to the hospital for low blood pressure/dehydration/mouth sores/urinary tract infection, fever, diarrhea, low WBC. Instruction: Neupogen for three days, further hydration, antidiarrheals with Immodium and Lomotil as needed, okay to add octreotide if diarrhea uncontrollable with meds.

In the hospital I am wheeled in a bed, first to one place then to another, put in a machine or on a machine or am attached to a machine, slid in, slid out, wheeled along long hallways, put back in a bed.

One night I wake up and find my arms tied to each side of my bedrails.

I cry for help. I need to get to a bathroom but I am tied to the bed. "Untie me," I beg, but nurses pass by and ignored me. "Let me get to the bathroom," I cry. A nurse offers me a bedpan. I refuse it. I can see the glow of the bathroom light just a few feet from my bed. I have only one wild desire, to get to the toilet in that room. I pull one arm free, then I untie the other. I leap from the bed.

And I slip. Slip in what is coming involuntarily out of my body. I try to stand up, but I slip and slide.

The nurses cry out in horror. More than one of them has to capture me, hold me up, clean me up, clean me off, change my gown, change my bedding. They make me take a pill. Later I learn it is Haldol, a drug they give to psychotic patients. They tell me they thought I was trying to escape. But no, I just wanted to go to the bathroom like a human being.

"Water," I beg. "Give me water."

"You're getting hydrated through your IV," a nurse explains. "You don't need more fluid just now."

"I need water."

They leave me alone. Tied again to the bed.

Late at night, in a very cold room, a new nurse approaches me. "I'm Angela," she says. "Would you like a sleeping pill?"

"Oh yes, please. You are an angel. I am so cold. I am so cold."

The nurse brings me two warm blankets; she presses them around my body. She unties my hands. She gives me water. "Now you will be warm and you will sleep." She gives me a pill. I swallow the pill. She strokes my hair gently and then I sleep.

EIGHTEEN
THE DRUGGIE LIFE AND BALD AS A BEAN

A T HOME AGAIN, NOW WITH NEW sweatpants, dark blue, and a white tee shirt that the hospital issued when Joe came to take me home and discovered that I had no clothes at the hospital—he had taken them all home in a bag—I find myself weak and in pain. The pain is something new, something deep and powerful, deep in the bones of my thighs.

I've been given shots of Neupogen in the hospital, a medicine to encourage the bone marrow to make neutrophils, those white blood cells that arrive at the site of an infection within an hour and kill the invading germs. My chemo has killed my killer cells, and neutropenia is the result. I have nothing with which to fight infection in my bloodstream.

Neupogen is going to fix that. Except there is a problem: the side effect is severe bone pain in my thighs. The activity going on in the marrow of my bones was so exceptional (I could picture great piles of white blood cells piling up and hitting the confines of the tunnel inside my bones) that the result is this awful, grinding pain.

I have drugs. I have Vicodin. I can take it every four to six hours around the clock. It is an opioid drug, it is strong, and it will help me escape the pain and allow me to sleep.

But in the morning, I have to eat something first. I hate eating now—food tastes all wrong, and the ulcers in my mouth resist food, reject food. My stomach, should food get to it, wants to send it back. I have already lost ten pounds.

Joe offers tea, toast, canned soup—that is about the limit of his culinary arts—but I have a memory of my mother's last days when she could not eat, before she was put on a feeding tube: she existed on cans of some chocolate drink.

I send Joe to the drugstore and he comes back with a six-pack of a high calorie chocolate drink. I discover I can manage that. In the morning, when my leg pain is extreme, I swallow that drink. I hold the cold plastic bottle in my hand, and I think, "Swallow. Then you get the pill. Then relief."

I begin to understand the yearnings of drug addicts. In a minute this pain will vanish and I will get relief. I will float above my anguish and pain and I will be saved.

First, chocolate drink. Then Vicodin. Then an hour later (it takes that long), the pain recedes, and I can find my way into life again.

This is indeed "the new reality," this life during chemo. I stay in bed most of the day. I don't want to talk. I don't want to watch television. I have no interest in reading. Or writing. I write nothing down, not one word.

I count the hours to my next pill. I call the special chemo pharmacist number and speak to one of the young Chinese pharmacists.

"I'm addicted," I tell her. "I'm a drug addict."

"No, no," she assures me. "Merrill, take the drugs you need. Take the Zofran before you become nauseated. Take the Ativan for anxiety. Take the Vicodin for pain. Merrill, you are on chemo. You are not a drug addict. You need these medicines to help you get through it. And when chemo is over, and when these symptoms recede, you simply won't want these drugs anymore."

"Yes, I will," I say. "I will want them forever."

"Then we'll help you get off them. Don't worry. And one more thing: don't eat your favorite foods during this period. They won't be your favorites anymore."

* * *

TWO WEEKS AFTER MY FIRST CHEMO (the only one so far), and right on schedule, I pull gently on my hair and a clump painlessly falls into my palm. I am calm about this development. It is a minor inconvenience, it was predicted (just as in my girlhood, the arrival of my breasts and menstruation were predicted). It is expected; it is something to which I have been looking forward.

I don't rush out to have my head shaved, as some in my cancer support community have done. I want to savor this development. I want to watch it happen and look in the mirror and see myself becoming bald. I have cancer, I'm on chemo, I'm going bald. It is a little mantra I can say to myself as I lie in bed and wonder how to pass the time. The nature of time has changed. There is now … and nothing else. There is pain to fight, there is hunger to invite. In addition to the chocolate drink, I am able to swallow a few slices of canned peaches. They slide down my throat as if they are live swimming fish. Joe eats alone in the kitchen since I cannot bear the smell of canned tomato soup or canned chili, the foods he mostly lives on.

On Thursday night, a week after I am home from the hospital, we go to the Cancer Support Center, Joe to the Caretaker Group, and I to the Cancer Patient Group. My daughter has sent me a pack of colored caps. I wear the pink cap. The breast-cancer-pink cap.

I am welcomed back, like a soldier returning from war. My friends are there, sitting on the soft couches, the soft chairs. One beautiful young woman cuddles into a knitted pink blanket. Lilly is her name. She has ovarian cancer. She says she can feel the cancer growing in there, like little fingers moving in her gut.

I don't have to tell my story anew—they know exactly where I have been. I tell them what I remember about my hospital stay ("I was tied to the bed!") and describe my pain ("My thighs feel as if they will explode!") I listen to their stories: the woman who has vaginal and cervical cancer and had to be in a radiation-proof room for four days while a radiation bullet was inserted in her body. The man with prostate cancer who is undergoing radiation treatments and hormonal treatments. The eighty-three-year-old woman whose breast cancer has returned as a new cancer. "I'm eighty-three, so I'll die of cancer. I have to die of something, don't I?" We laugh. The concept of sex is discussed. "Sex? Who can even remember it!" The man taking hormone treatments tells us his girlfriend is getting frustrated. We laugh. We laugh a lot in our group. I tell them I am a drug addict and they laugh with me. What fun we are having. I feel a bit of happiness here. Our leader is great fun herself—she says that since having breast reconstruction, she could walk smack into a brick wall, chest first, and feel no pain. Laughter. We spend time discussing how bad doctors can be. Male doctors! Another woman with breast cancer has undergone reconstructive surgery. She told her surgeon she wanted "new girls, a small size" and the surgeon gave her size D-cup breasts. He couldn't imagine she wouldn't be grateful—she was still so young and pretty. She has to see him again to have him tattoo nipples onto her breasts. She doesn't trust him now. What else might he decide to decorate her with?

What fun we have at Group. When our time is up, we embrace one another in a circle as we have done since the first meeting. We wish each other health, blessings, a week ahead in which to enjoy the life we have. One woman announces she will hold us all in her prayers. It doesn't seem a bad idea. I welcome the thought. I consider praying myself, though I have no idea how to do it. Prayer seems to bring deep comfort to some. I think perhaps I will pray to my father. He is long dead; he died of leukemia when he was just fifty-six. He always wore a gold horseshoe ring, with the U-shape turned up so the luck would never run out. But his luck did run out. He is up there floating in the land of the dead—some of my praying friends have assured me of this. He is watching over me, looking after me, and he is as dear to me as God the Father is to some others. I can pray to him. I can say, "Daddy, I love you so much. Daddy, I hope you are with Mommy. You and Mommy are on my wall in your wedding picture. Daddy, I miss you. Daddy, I have cancer, like you. But Daddy, don't worry. I'm too old to die young."

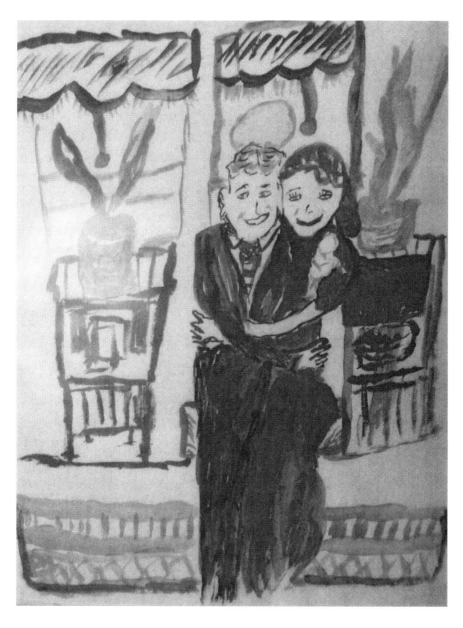

Mom and Dad's wedding painting

NINETEEN
LOOK GOOD, FEEL BETTER—
FACE-OFF AT THE 7-ELEVEN

❦

I NEITHER LOOK GOOD NOR FEEL BETTER but this is about to change. After I attend this special workshop for cancer patients, I am assured a new confidence will result. A makeup artist "to the stars" is going to distribute samples of high end cosmetics and show us how to apply them.

We meet in a room with eight women, half of whom are bravely bald—no hats, no scarves. I am only half bald, having lost chunks of hair with the passing days, so I am wearing one of the caps my daughter sent me.

We are asked only one question as we come into the room: is our skin color fair, olive, or dark? We are then given a little red carry bag, its contents adapted to our coloring, of lip liner, lipstick, blush, eye shadow, concealer, mascara, foundation, powder—the name brands you might see advertised in *Vogue*. Not that I read *Vogue*, unless I am in the dentist's office.

We begin with eyebrow pencil. Our instructor indicates the angles that one's eyebrows should take—something I have never considered, having accepted the eyebrows I was born with. There is some discussion of eyebrow plucking, eyebrow threading, eyebrow tattooing .... We are busy opening little tubes and packages and boxes and sticks of various colors and sizes. We each have a mirror, and we are urged to try everything on our faces.

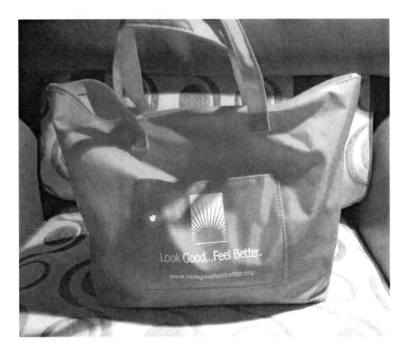

Look Good, Feel Better

I remember when my daughters were in college—ardent feminism was their standard—how the many issues of makeup, hair dying, leg shaving, and ear piercing were discussed at home.

I began coloring my hair at about age thirty-eight. I know it was partly a reaction to my own mother's going gray in her thirties and how friends sometimes mistook her for my grandmother. My hair never required a beauty salon. My aunt had run a small beauty shop in our Brooklyn house, and I learned early how to cut hair. I always cut my own. My choice of hair dye was "medium brown" Colorsilk. There were some rumors about hair dye possibly causing cancer, but no one could prove it. I knew it would be difficult to quit dying my hair and to weather the awkward growing-out period. Now, of course, there was no question of a growing-out period. There was just the falling-out period.

We have an instructive and entertaining hour looking at our new beauty aids and learning how to use them. "If you don't use them all, they make great Christmas presents!" our teacher tells us. At the end of the hour we have a surprise—a door is opened to a small room containing dozens of wigs and hats and scarves. We are invited to try them on. We are invited to choose one in any of the many styles and colors to take home with us.

Most all of the wigs are outrageously wildly curly or spiky, or pink and purple, or long, sexy blonde … but they are here only for fun, not as serious wigs. A serious wig, the kind that might look the way our hair used to look, is offered to us free by the American Cancer Society. We are given a number to call to make an appointment to get the real thing—a wig that will remind us of what we used to call our hair.

But today I choose a long blonde wig to take home. Then I call my sister, Bobbie. She invites me to come over. Here we are that day:

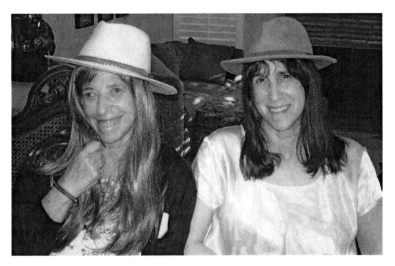

Merrill in wig with sister

A week later I call and make an appointment at the "free wig" office of the American Cancer Society. My daughter Becky will take some time off from work at the library and drive me there.

"You should eat something," Joe says. "Don't go without eating something."

His advice sounds to me like, "You should climb a mountain before you go. Don't go without climbing a mountain."

I look in the cabinet for some sliced peaches. We are out of them. Who is shopping these days? I am finding cans in the cabinet that expired in 1980. I poke around some cans of pickled beets, some jars of borscht—why was I into beets in a big way? I find two small cans of green chilis—I once made enchiladas—some boxes of instant mashed potatoes, and a can of crushed pineapple that is so swollen it is about to explode and spray botulism all over the kitchen.

"Eat something, eat anything," Joe urges me. I find one tiny jar of Mandarin orange segments and open it. Any food I eat has to have its own sliding capacity—a wet, small item that can slide down my throat with the least contact against the ulcers still in my mouth. (The "magic mouthwash" is of no use; it is thick and pink and smells like Pepto-Bismol. Just the sight of it makes me nauseated.) But the orange pieces go down my throat like children careening down a waterslide. Willy-nilly the food gets into me.

Becky picks me up, and we drive off toward the east on the freeway. The San Gabriel Mountains to the north glow in the noontime sunshine. Big puffy clouds draw pictures of animals in the sky. I breathe deeply. I'm out here is the world, with birds and flowers and majestic pine trees dotting the mountaintops. It has been so long since I've noticed any of the beauties of nature. Where have I been? I've been in chemo! Now I am in my third week. Dr. B has removed the ultra-poisonous drug from the cocktail that has nearly killed me and I am now on only two drugs, Taxol and Herceptin.

Still, as we drive along, I realize that perhaps it was a major mistake to go on a trip that takes me more than ten feet from a bathroom. Despite my anti-nausea drugs and the Vicodin I've already taken this morning for pain, I sense my Mandarin orange segments are suddenly moving upward.

"Becky, I need a bathroom. Can you find me someplace fast?"

My daughter exits the freeway, speeds toward a populated street, and within a block we see a 7-Eleven on a corner. She screeches into the parking lot. She rushes into the store with me.

"Where is your restroom, please?" my daughter asks. The

owner, wearing a Sikh turban, says, "Sorry, we have no public restrooms here."

Becky, normally shy and soft-spoken, walks up to face the man: "My mother has cancer. My mother is taking chemotherapy. My mother has to throw up. We know you have a bathroom here. Show it to us."

The man's mouth falls open. He says nothing. He points behind some shelves of Coke. I stumble down a hallway, find a filthy bathroom, a dirty sink, and gratefully make use of it. I shock myself by looking in the mirror. Who is that woman, hairless— my scarf has fallen off my head—pale, shaken? Is another wave of nausea rising? It certainly doesn't smell too good in the room. I look around for bleach to clean the sink. There is none, nor is there soap in the soap dispenser. I wait to see if I need to throw up again. It seems I don't. I decide that Mandarin oranges are now off the menu for the rest of my life.

I set my expression to neutral and get out of there. My daughter awaits me among the aisles of Red Bull and packaged donuts.

"Thank you so much," I say to the bearded man who stands baffled and confused, wearing his twisted turban.

Becky follows me out of the store.

"Thank you," I say to her. "That was very brave of you."

"You're the brave one, Mom. How do you feel?"

"I feel just fine now. Let's move on to discover my new head of hair."

WE PARK IN THE LOT OF a small private hospital, beautifully landscaped, with the backdrop of the mountains in the distance. The waiting area is furnished like a lovely home—soft thick carpets, flowered couches, vases of roses and lilies.

I peer into a room and see a woman apparently getting a chemo infusion—the machinery is the same as at my hospital—but she and her companion are in a private cozy corner. I wonder how one manages to be treated here for cancer. Is there an audition necessary, an entry exam?

We ask the receptionist about the wig room and are directed

down a softly lit hallway featuring modern art on its walls. Inside is a welcoming woman who invites me to sit in a chair in front of a mirror and motions to the towering piles of wigs on shelves, even on windowsills, all around the room.

"But first," she says, "you'll have to wear this little net thing." It looks like the toe end of panty hose, the kind of mask criminals pull over their faces before they rob a bank. She removes the scarf from my head, exposing the pathetic image of my skull, not totally hairless yet, for there are a few stray strands hanging on—a sight I'd like to spare even my daughter. Then the woman puts the tight, awful robber's mask over my scalp. I am already feeling nauseated again.

"So what sort of hairpiece are you looking for, dear?"

"I used to have short curly brown hair," I say.

"Oh my, I don't know if we have anything like that. We have lots of long hair, and lots of blonde hair, and some very attractive jet-black wigs. But let me look."

She begins to poke among the plastic packages housing the wigs, tossing some to one side, some to the other. Becky watches her hunting, unsuccessfully, for a short, curly, brown-haired wig.

"What you need is a wig librarian," my librarian daughter says to her. "These wigs need to be catalogued. They should be in some kind of order."

"Let's try this nice one," the woman says. But the thing she puts over the tighter thing on my head is monstrous. Tufts of black hair stick up around my face as if I've been struck by lightning.

"Excuse me," I ask, "but is there a restroom nearby?"

"Oh dear, yes, down the hall, but you can't go running out with that wig on your head."

"Well," I reply, leaping out of the chair, "I can't go running down the hall without it."

I escape, rushing through the carpeted hallways till I find a women's room.

This time it isn't nausea, I realize, but violent stomach cramps. I find a toilet just in time.

"Oh, God."

I must have spoken out loud, because a woman's voice asks me, "Honey, are you okay?"

"I'm on chemo."

"Me, too," she says. "I know the script. Can I help you in any way?"

"I'll be right out."

When the fury passes, I stand up and the toilet flushes on its own.

We two women are at the sink washing our hands. "I came here to get a wig," I explain.

"I gave up on them," she says, "but I like these pretty scarves. I've learned how to twist and tie them. You can look online and learn how to do it."

"I've got to get back and get this thing off my head."

"I know. Wigs feel like tight earmuffs. I know exactly what it's like."

"Good luck to you," I tell her.

"Let's live and be well," she says, and we turn to each other and hug.

People with cancer know how much a hug means.

Back in the wig room, Becky has apparently been helping the woman find a few brown wigs. I pull off the one on my head, and Becky helps the woman place the next one.

"Fine! This one is absolutely perfect," I say. "I adore it, it's the real me, let's take it. I'm so grateful. Thank you for your help. We really must be going now. We've got to rush home before the traffic gets heavy."

And we escape.

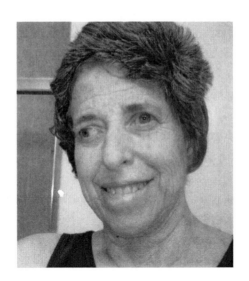

Funny wig

TWENTY
MY JEWISH BOOK CLUB

BEFORE I LEARNED I HAD BREAST cancer, I belonged to a Jewish book club. Eight Jewish women meeting for forty years, once a month in one of our houses.

Did we ever read a book? Who knows? Did we ever discuss a book? We had arguments every time:

"Why should I read a historical novel when I'm not interested in historical novels?"

"Then why should I read a book about how Yiddish is coming back from a lost language when my grandparents only wanted that it should *be* a lost language?"

"They told secrets in my house in Yiddish so the kids wouldn't know what they were talking about."

"I think next month we should read a modern romance novel. There's a new one on the bestseller list."

"I'm against reading bestsellers. They're crap."

"I'm too old for romance. I can't be bothered with romance."

"Molly, you've had three husbands. How did you manage that without romance?"

"Look at my breasts! They speak for themselves. Also I'm a good cook."

"Could it be your cooking poisoned the first two?"

"Funny that is not."

"Sex must figure in somewhere."

"If it figures, it figures. Remember how in *Fiddler on the Roof*, Tevye sings, 'Do you love me?' and his wife answers, 'For twenty-five years I've cooked your meals, washed your clothes, shared your bed .... If that isn't love, what is?' "

"It's your bosoms, it's not your cooking, that got you three husbands."

"They should live and be well," Molly said, patting her bosoms lovingly. "But you never know. One in eight women gets breast cancer. It could be one of us."

"Never one of us. We're not the type."

We are the type, in fact. We are especially the type. Women with Ashkenazic genetics are especially at risk. If we carry the Braca gene mutation, we have an eighty-five percent risk of being diagnosed with cancer in our lifetime, and are also at high risk for ovarian cancer.

Sprinkled over the years among our discussions of life and literature were exchanges of really important information. Who were the best pediatricians? Orthodontists? The best summer camps for the kids? When busing started in our city, most of the neighborhood children were pulled out and put into Christian or Catholic private schools. And since all of us in our book club had been educated in the public schools of New York—the Bronx or Brooklyn—we strongly resisted private schools. Pay for schools? Ridiculous! Didn't we all feel grateful for our public school educations? And look how smart we were?

Smart we were. There was no argument there.

We and our husbands had all bought houses in our Southern California neighborhood in the late sixties. When our children were young, we stayed home and raised them. Our husbands were out there in the world doing something respectable—being teachers or engineers or working for Xerox or the Jet Propulsion Lab. But when the children were older, all of us women went back to school and finished our degrees if we hadn't already done so. We went to work. Teaching.

How come we continued to call our group a book club when

we practically never read the same book? We fought each other at every meeting. Why not read about gardening, about art? Why not read the novels of Philip Roth? All the women but me claimed they were disgusted by Philip Roth's books.

"Such a dirty mind."

"Such a dirty mouth!"

"What he did to that piece of liver!"

"You didn't have to read it, did you?"

"Such an honest writer," I said. "He proves that our crazy Jewish relatives are worthy subjects for great literature." I was already a writer myself when I told them that. I was already writing about my own relatives. I had discovered a gold mine in the characters of my family, with Roth's books as my guide.

I thought Philip Roth could lead us all openly into the land of sex. If we read *Portnoy's Complaint,* we could talk about sex, about sex in marriage—so far as I knew, the only kind we had—about how we viewed sex, felt about sex. We talked about everything else. Why not sex?

"I don't talk in public about such things," Shelly announced. The other women concurred.

"Let's not rock the boat."

Sickness we could talk about, not about sex.

Being overweight we could talk about, not about sex.

Having trouble with the children we could talk about.

We all loved this joke.

> A group of women meets one afternoon.
> 'Oy,' says the first woman.
> 'Oy vey,' says the second woman.
> 'Oy vey is mir,' says the third woman.
> 'Ladies, ladies,' says the fourth woman. 'We promised we wouldn't talk about our children!'

Much laughter, then the coffee cake.

Sometimes just coffee cake. But if we met for lunch, as we often did, then one of us cooked noodle pudding or matzo ball soup or kasha and brisket and *then* we had the coffee cake. Such a bond we had, but it had nothing to do with books. It had to do with growing up in Brooklyn or the Bronx, with having had the parents and grandparents we had, for being alive because our Jewish grandparents hadn't stayed in Poland or Germany, but got out. What really connected us was talking about wallpaper and remodeling our kitchens and observing one another's jewelry and admiring it. We inspected the new couch and chair one of us had and discussed how good a buy it was. We compared the children's achievements (none of them had yet become depressed or bipolar or drug-addicted or worst of all, fallen in love with a non-Jew). We discussed piano lessons, violin lessons, more piano lessons. And lawyers, should we need one. Who were the good ones? Who were the Jewish ones? Which lawyers also belonged to the synagogue? I was the only one of us who didn't belong to the synagogue.

And then we heard that Eileen Schwartzman, who belonged to the synagogue, had cancer. Breast cancer. She was only forty-three and she was dying.

"One in eight women gets breast cancer," Myrna said.

"That means one of *us* will get it," said Helen.

"It won't be one of us. It doesn't run in our families." We had already ascertained how each of our mothers, if they were dead, had died. As we got older, every one of our mothers had died. None died from breast cancer.

Myrna's mother fell and broke her hip when she was eighty-five and didn't want to be helpless. She refused to go to a nursing home. One night she called all her daughters to her bedside. On her bed she had her big jewelry box.

Myrna's mother dangled a necklace. "Which one of you wants this really gorgeous one?" She dangled a pair of earrings. "Who would kill to get this pair?" She held her biggest diamond ring up to the light. "Which one of you would be willing to poison me for this one?"

Myrna's mother wasn't kidding. The night after she distributed all her jewelry, all her gold, all her diamonds, all her award pins from Hunter High School, that very night after her daughters had gone home and after the hired aide had fallen asleep, she swallowed the contents of a bottle of sleeping pills and for good measure, wrapped a plastic bag around her neck, fastening it firmly with a thick rubber band.

"She was so brave," Myrna told us proudly at the funeral. "I admire her so much. I hope I have the guts to do it when my time comes."

SOMETHING HAPPENED THAT RUINED THE BOOK club for me. On that day, I walked out of Molly's house, never to return. We were meeting in the thick of summer. Though Molly had known for a month the book club was meeting at her house, she had, for some reason, decided to have her cleaning lady to the house on that day. The maid was running the vacuum cleaner in the next room, and it roared in our ears. The maid was listening to Mexican music on the radio—*blasting* salsa music.

"Molly," I said, "how are we going to have our book club meeting with all this noise?"

"I decided today we would meet outside. We're having company this weekend and I needed the house cleaned."

"Outside? It's one hundred degrees outside."

"I'm making plenty of iced tea."

I looked out into the backyard, where Molly had a chicken coop in the corner of her yard. She raised hens so she could collect free eggs every day. Flies abounded out there, along with the smell of chicken shit.

I sat there on her couch with my purse in my lap, wondering if she could possibly mean that we were going to sit outside in the sun, eat our lunches in the sun. Did the other women see that this would be impossible? They were already noshing on nuts and raisins that Molly had set out on the coffee table.

I opened my purse to see if I had sunglasses with me. I did, but what the hell, I was not going to sit out there in the blazing heat because she felt it was convenient to have her cleaning lady come that day. I put my purse down on her coffee table in front of the couch. Next to the bowl of nuts.

Molly yelled: "Get that purse off my table! God knows where it's been. It could have all kinds of germs on it.'"

I had been to Molly's house dozens of times. I had put my purse on her coffee table dozens of times. Suddenly my purse had become a death-dealing instrument of terror?

The vacuum cleaner continued to roar. The salsa music blasted in my ears. I got up from Molly's couch, I took my filthy purse off her table, and I left her house. For good.

I left her house, I left my Jewish book club forever. I left my friends in it—What friends? All they did was argue and compare jewelry—and I freed myself from the endless round of never discussing books, from the stupidity of women who were too obtuse to read and love Philip Roth, from the obligatory cleaning up of my house on book club day, of putting bleach in the toilet, and of cooking a meal for them. For these women I would cook no more meals. For ungrateful Molly, I would simmer no more prunes for the *tzimmes*.

But when word got around, a year later, that I had breast cancer, I found a plastic grocery bag in my mailbox. In it was a crocheted cap made of green cotton. The note from Molly said: "Merrill, so your head shouldn't be cold at night."

TWENTY-ONE
FREE LUXURY APARTMENT IN HOLLYWOOD!

THE NEXT STEP—AND THERE'S ALWAYS A next step with breast cancer—is to confer with a radiologist about radiation treatment. Joe and I go to the facility on Sunset Boulevard and meet Dr. Goy, who in spite of his name, which might give a Jewish girl pause, is a handsome, kind Asian doctor.

He examines me and has good news. Because of my incredible luck in having relatively small breasts, I will need only four weeks of radiation, not six. We are taken to another room where I have a CT scan taken, where Dr. Goy draws blue circles on my breast with his marker pen, and where a dosimetrist, the specialist who calculates the distribution and the angles of radiation, will make his assessment. Dr. Goy tells me that at my first radiation treatment the nurse will make some small tattoos that look like freckles on my breast. I have the thought that Orthodox Jews cannot be tattooed—but then again, I am not Orthodox.

After the doctor has finished drawing on my breast, he and the dosimetrist disappear into a little room to do their elaborate calculations. The idea is to radiate as little healthy tissue as possible, to avoid radiating my heart—in my case, my heart happens to be in the line of fire behind my left breast—and to do as little damage as possible, so that my ribs won't crack at some future sneeze, and a new cancer won't be initiated by the radiation. At the end of the four weeks of radiation, there will be an extra "boost" of radiation given to the area of the scar and then I will be all done.

There's a problem, though. My HMO has only two sites that do radiation treatment. One is in Ontario, thirty miles from home but the route is on freeways. The other is right here on Sunset Boulevard in Hollywood, a few miles closer to our home but on heavily trafficked roads.

Joe and I discuss with Dr. Goy the coming days of required excessive travel. But wait ... he has an amazing offer for us. The HMO will give us a free apartment just a half block from this building. We can live there for the month I am having radiation treatment. This is now calculated to begin at the start of September.

"Take a look at the apartments," Dr. Goy urges us. "They have everything you will need."

At first I am elated. A free month in the center of Movieland. All meals in restaurants. No laundry, no shopping, no cooking. A little honeymoon, if you like. And with only the slight inconvenience of, once a day, lying down in a linear accelerator for about five minutes and having burning rays directed into my breast.

We take the address of the free place and walk over to see it. It's a perfectly nice apartment building from an older time, and a perfectly kind young woman takes us up in an elevator along with another couple, one of whom is also going to need a long period of radiation. We're given the key to one of the apartments.

Inside, we look around and then we look at each other. This is just fine, we remark to each other; it's even better than our attic apartment in Cambridge, Massachusetts, where we lived just after we got married. But no, what could be better than that first apartment, where the ceiling slanted so deeply in the bathroom that we two, in the shower together, had to duck our heads?

There's a bedroom (two single beds), a living room (a fifties couch, a coffee table, and an old model TV), a bathroom (I don't even look in there), and a tiny kitchen with a small wooden table and two chairs. We'd have to bring our own dishes, linens, and bedsheets.

A month of imprisonment is what we both see at the same

instant. My treatment, and then a walk back here to wait for the next day's treatment. Radiation is not a honeymoon: I will be fatigued, I will be burned, I will be needing lots of sleep. We will not be touring the homes of the movie stars, we will not be visiting the Modern Art Museum, we will not be trying out all the bistros and cafés or dancing at the clubs every night.

At home, let us admit it, we have all the comforts of home. We have adjoining adjustable beds with memory foam mattresses. We have a kitchen window that looks out on my bird feeders. If we leave for a month, all our hummingbirds and chickadees will starve. We have not one but two computers. And we have Joe's grand piano. How could he possibly imagine being without his piano, his Bach, his Beethoven, his Mendelssohn, for four weeks?

How can we live without email, without Google, without Yahoo?

On the way out, after returning the key, we ask the young woman how one might use a computer here. She says there is this hospital library several blocks away where one can get a Wi-Fi signal.

Never mind; we will go home right now to our nice house with a front yard, a backyard, a soft couch, and all the Wi-Fi one could desire. When it's time for my radiation, we will drive to Ontario, which I have heard is the hotspot in Southern California for cow farms. We will visit the cows.

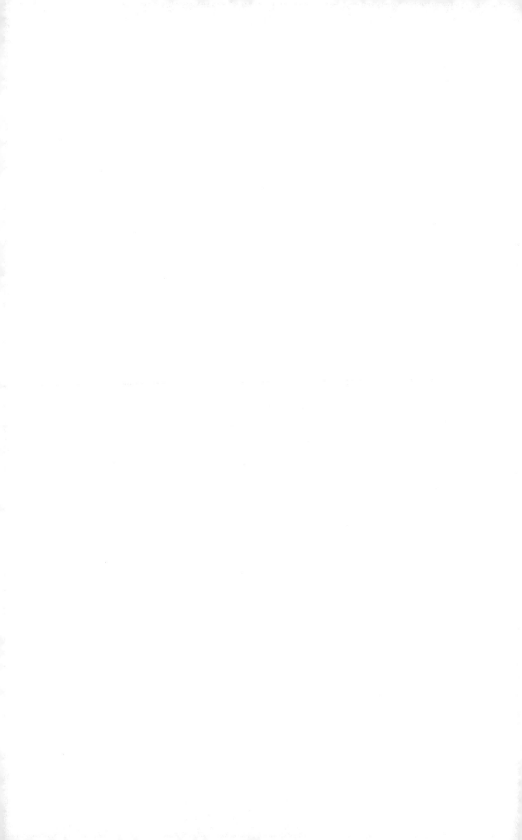

TWENTY-TWO
LILLY DIES

DEATH HAS COME TO OUR SUPPORT group. Lilly, the young, beautiful woman who could feel the fingers of her ovarian cancer moving in her belly, who could feel her cancer cells gorging themselves on her healthy cells, had gone back to the hospital for one more ultimate, last-hope, massive dose of chemotherapy.

To the email I write her, afterward, telling her we all miss her, we want her back, she replies, "Merrill dear, this chemo has kicked my ass."

Then: nothing. No Lilly at Group. No word. No news.

Fear. Others in the group are also failing: the tall man in the cowboy hat and boots whose last wish was to go to the county fair and watch the pig races. The very young mother with two small children—brain cancer. The flight attendant, now seventy, who refuses to believe that she, who exercises, who eats only salads, has breast cancer. She came just once, but never again. The startlingly beautiful black woman who amazes us with the news that she has lost 150 pounds due to naso-pharyngeal cancer—and there she is at group, with a perfect figure.

Two speakers come to the cancer center—one discussing the benefits and blessings of hospice care, which we are not up to yet, and one who calls his talk "The Boogie Man in the Closet."

Joe and I come to the Cancer Support Center to listen to his talk, but it seems to me the man is writing lecture notes on a blackboard in cloud formations. What is he saying? What does he mean? Get used to death? Don't fear death? Why is he telling stories about his mother, who died young? What can he teach us? How can he reassure us? He can't. He doesn't. One woman, not in our group but frail with the chill of severe illness written on her face, suddenly gets up and leaves. I draw little Jewish stars on the paper in my lap—there is no possible justification for not being terrified of the Boogie Man in the Closet. He wants from us what we most want to keep. I draw a sketch of the closet. I draw the image of the Boogie Man in the Closet, and then I bolt that closet door. I draw ten locking bolts on that closet door. *Deadbolts.*

On the table at the back of the room is a jar of apple juice and a box of cookies. I get up and pour a glass of juice and grab some cookies. I walk out of the room and go sit on a soft couch in the entry area. I read a magazine called *Cure.* Moments later, Joe comes looking for me.

"Let's get out of here. I've had enough."

"Me, too. Shall we go out to dinner?"

Dinner, any meal in fact, is still a great problem for me. Though my chemo cocktail is now only Herceptin—the antibody for the aggressive HER 2 neu factor in my breast cancer—I still have no interest in food. It all tastes like the inside lid of a tin can. I have by now lost thirty pounds and rather appreciate the improvement in every way—in my knees, which have less weight to carry, and in my wardrobe: my good-looking silk pants now fit me very nicely.

Joe pulls in at China Café. "Let's try this place," he says. "I like these small places, a Chinese family cooking in the back, mainly a take-out business."

The woman at the desk looks at the scarf wrapped around my head and holds up her hand to indicate she will be right back. She returns carrying a bowl of egg drop soup.

"Sit," she indicates. "My daughter also has this sickness. But can swallow this soup."

And there, in the warm broth, swirling with little ribbons of cooked egg, I find a food I can eat and actually enjoy. For the first time since beginning chemo, I feel a thrill in swallowing something warm and delicious, steaming and precious. There is protein here, and a few swimming peas and thin mushrooms. I can swallow this. I feel hunger. I feel gratitude. I want to offer thanks to the powers that allow me to live on.

Joe's dish is a savory fish in black bean sauce. He seems to relish every bite. When we leave, we order two take-out containers of egg drop soup. The kind woman at the desk adds a dozen free fortune cookies to the bag. "You get well," she says. I could have kissed her. I did, in fact, touch her cheek gently with my hand.

Lilly has died. We get word in Group that there will be a memorial service at a home in the hills. An address is given, and a time. Beautiful Lilly. Young, vibrant, as pretty as a young woman could be, sensual, sexy, witty, funny, intelligent, in love with a handsome jazz musician, her ass kicked and her voice stilled. Dead.

How does death really happen? What are the steps, inch by inch? And so fast? How do we perceive the mystery of the passage from being alive to not being at all? At Group we ponder how you go from something as big and alive and aware as each of us is to … nothing. To an entity turned off, empty, motionless, vacant, limp. Disappeared. Gone and gone forever.

My father in his coffin, my mother in hers. Effigies, puppets, bad art made by third-rate artists, my mother's lips sewn together, my father's mustache carelessly shaved off, his falsely suntanned skin making him into a cartoon of the man he was. My mother's lips colored with red—never! Their hands, which I lifted and then dropped: heavy as lead, cold as doom.

Just last week I found a rat floating dead in the pool … swollen near to bursting with decomposing gasses, an animal stinking and dead.

"Burn me fast," I tell Joe later that night. "Grind up my bones, I don't mind. But I don't want to rot."

At Lilly's memorial, there is sunshine, music, a patio strewn with fragrant flowers, and at the door, a collage of the usual representations of a life: the fun times, school pictures, high school prom pictures, and friends, the family, and centrally, the lovely dead girl.

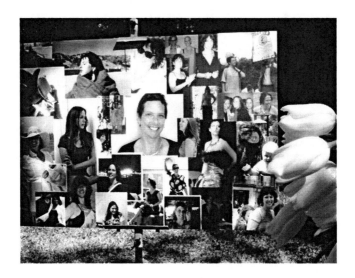

Lilly's memorial service

Inside the house we find furniture hand-carved from the trunks of great trees. We are in an artist's den, every surface smooth, shined to perfection, redolent of the deep woods. And on every table—food, drink, sweets.

Lilly's lover is putting sandwiches together in the kitchen—a handsome, tall, powerhouse of a man, holding up under whatever onslaught of pain is beneath the surface. Lilly's sister and Lilly's mother are close behind him, touching him, touching each other.

And who are all these children? Nieces, nephews, cousins? Lilly had not yet had children. She wanted children, she adored children. The parts of her body that were to make children turned into her killer. How upside down, how wrong.

We, from the Cancer Support Group, learn more of Lilly's life from those who loved and knew her so well. Friends tell stories about her. They sob, remembering shared adventures. Tears and more tears fall. We in our group, the six of us who have become good friends, wonder if we should speak too. And yes, why not?

One by one, we go up to the front of the group, stand under the garlands of hung flowers, and remember her, each in our own way—her wit, her jokes, her irony, the comfort of her simple charming sweet self in the room with us, a glimmering soul.

That morning, I read in the paper about the death of a famous Polish poet, *Wislawa Szymborska,* who, born in 1923, died at eighty-nine. She died in her sleep—an end she anticipated in a poem published fifty-four years earlier called "I'm Working on the World." This is the poem I choose to read at Lilly's memorial service. In this poem we are told that death will come in sleep, that we will dream that breathing isn't necessary. We won't feel terror any more than we would at the sound of falling petals.

TWENTY-THREE
PINK GIFTS

M Y KIND FRIENDS WISH TO DISTRACT me from cancer. One brings me a pink bracelet made of parachute strands, strong enough that if unwound they could hold me up for a week over the Grand Canyon. The bracelet is so heavy and thick, I imagine this is exactly the way handcuffs feel. Besides, I already have a pink bracelet that says on it: "Left hand, no needles, no BP." I am not lacking for cancer jewelry.

A neighbor from across the street arrives with a pink hydrangea plant.

My sister's son and his wife give me a pink frying pan, made in Italy and guaranteed, by its purchase, to help in the battle against breast cancer. It's a pretty pot, for a pot, but the idea of cooking in it is disabling for me. Stewing, frying, burning in a cancer pot. I put it at the very back of my pot cabinet. Perhaps, after my treatment is finished, I will consider using it.

My dear friend Nancy, who'd had not one siege of breast cancer, but two, one of them a mastectomy, sends me a pink singing doll.

When I press the button on the doll's hand, its mouth begins to open and close and a song comes flying out. It is "I hope you dance," by Lee Ann Womack. All about love and hope and joy and hunger for life.

When my children visit, I want to give the doll to one of my granddaughters, but their mothers do not want either of them to have a singing cancer doll.

A meditation tape arrives from my dear elementary school friend, Barbara—the girl who took me to see Charlton Heston's apartment in Hell's Kitchen on my thirteenth birthday, just after we had seen him in the movie *The Greatest Show On Earth*. At the very instant we were reading, in awe, his name on the mailbox, he drove up in a big cream-colored Packard and said, "What can I do for you girls?" My friend told him it was my birthday, and could she take a picture of me with him? He said, "Well, of course, I'd be honored," and he put his arm around me and she took the picture. It came out blurry, but I still have it and I love it. He wasn't big on guns at that time.

I try out the meditation CD one day as I lie in bed. I play it on an old portable CD player, with earphones over my ears. The female voice is gentle and sweet, with just a touch of a foreign accent, and she informs me that I am a vessel with two openings, one at the top of my head and one in the soles of my feet. In the hole at the top of my head, God, as a brilliant light (choose your own favorite color) is expanding to fill every cell of my being.

Below, from the soles of my feet, muddy water is being pushed out, all toxins, cancer cells, poisons from my treatment, all worries, angers, frustrations and fears. The brilliant light (I choose the color aqua) is now making its home in my body, healing me, nurturing me, and giving me energy.

I am paying attention but am beginning to worry about where the muddy water is draining out. This bed is expensive—it is adjustable, and it has a memory foam mattress.

I skip to the next exercise on the CD, and this puts me at the side of a beautiful lake on a moonlit night. I am to think of the number 9, which is the magic healing number in Oriental medicine. Breathe deeply, it tells me, inhale the feminine nurturing energy of the moonlight. It will heal my scar tissue, my burned body, enter every cell.

Now I must picture a loved one serving me an elegant glass

filled with moonlight. It is soft, feminine, the essence of sunshine as well.

The third guided meditation begins by asking me to name my heart's desire. I must imagine my eyes glowing, my heart aflame. They get brighter whenever I breathe. I must speak my heart's desire aloud. All this visualizing will fill me with peace, define my "truth."

Just as I am wondering about my heart's desire, I am told that my eyes are like warm stones in sand. I must become aware of my ears, my throat, my face, all peaceful and relaxed.

The phone rings. I jerk and try to reach for it. My hand becomes tangled in the wires of the earphones connected to the CD player. I answer the phone and a recorded voice warns me that the FBI says there is a robbery once every thirty seconds in my neighborhood. That a break-in could be occurring now at my very front door. That life in these times is extremely dangerous.

TWENTY-FOUR
WE'RE GOING ON A TRIP
IN OUR FAVORITE ROCKET SHIP

THIS SUMMER, ACCORDING TO JEWISH LAW, my eldest grandson will become a man. His Bar Mitzvah is planned in Washington, DC—but will I be able to take the trip? I confer with Dr. B. She has decided to continue treating me with only one chemotherapy drug, Herceptin, which I now get every three weeks. She has news: in the fall they'll be moving the infusion department to a beautiful new site in the hospital building, overlooking a pond and a fountain.

She thinks I should take the trip. Yes, I'm bald, and yes, I'm very tired, but we'll time my infusions so that I'll have two weeks free from treatment, from doctors, from blood tests and from medical worries. My recent heart scan showed that so far Herceptin has not damaged my heart function, my ejection fraction is good, my red and white blood cells have good numbers, and the pains in my legs can still be treated with Vicodin if I need it.

We buy tickets on Jet Blue. Becky and her eleven-year-old son Jacob will also fly to DC from Los Angeles, but on another airline. We confer with our grandson's other grandparents, who live in Berlin; we decide we will all rent a comfortable house for two weeks and share it with Becky and Jacob. Our youngest daughter and her family will stay with her sister's family.

When I tell my youngest granddaughter on the phone that we

are going on a trip, that she too will be going on this trip, she begins to sing a song from her favorite TV show, *Little Einsteins*. I find myself singing this tune every day, many times a day: "We're going on a trip in our favorite rocket ship, zooming through the sky!" I'm excited. I plan my wardrobe; I plan my head-covering. I know that Orthodox Jewish women always wear head-coverings or the sheitel—wig. For Orthodox Jewish women, the uncovered head is a sign of immodesty or worse. Married Jewish women cover their heads so as not to attract other men.

I haven't attracted the attention of men for a long time. I feel considerable grief about this. A man might sometimes hold a door open for me at a store, but because I'm old, not because I'm attractive.

This might not be the best time to see the glass as half full, but in truth my toes are numb all the time, my fingernails crack and must be cut to the quick, my taste buds have not totally recovered, and my libido has flown the coop. Joe assures me it will all "come back," but I suspect he is mainly assuring himself. I try to cover my head when I go to bed. I wear the crocheted cap that Molly, from my book club, made for me, but usually during the night I fling it off. I ask Joe if it disturbs him, looking at my bald head, and he says it doesn't, not at all. It disturbs me. I look like another soul, not like myself. I look like an alien.

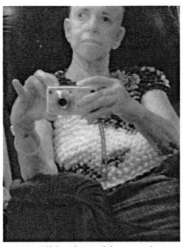

Merrill looking like an alien

I get busy, however, with making my trip list. There are all the usual things: stop the newspaper delivery, turn off the water supply to the washing machine, have the post office hold the mail, ask my sister's husband to water the tomato plants that our gardener has planted for me in the backyard, pack pills and shoes and underwear and presents for the grandchildren and for the other grandparents, and take my portable radio and my laptop computer and my cell phone and wires and plugs and chargers and what not.

Is this not really too much for me? Do I even want to go to a Bar Mitzvah? Did I give my own children any religious education? No, I did not. Do I think religion is the cause of terrible crimes and atrocities? Yes, I do. Do I know people with cancer who take tremendous comfort in being religious and praying to God? Yes, I do. Have I been told by friends that they are praying for me? Yes, I have. I have thanked them. Do I know people who are not afraid to die because God will receive them in his majestic empire in heaven? Of course I do.

But I don't have these comforts. I seem to think my mother once told me that when we die, we will all hold hands and fly to heaven together. But she couldn't have told me that. I took care of her in her last ten years of life when she was paralyzed by a stroke and on a feeding tube and not even able to turn herself over in bed and she never once talked about heaven. Not once.

How I miss my mother and father suddenly. I want to be back home in Brooklyn with them. I want to be at the Bronx Zoo with them, as I was when I was seven years old, holding a box of Cracker Jack.

But I can visit them only in my dreams, in the zoo of my dreams, in my stories, in my paintings. They have been dead so long now.

But it all plays forward. My grandson is going to become a man in August, and I am going to witness it. I am going on a trip in my favorite rocket ship.

* * *

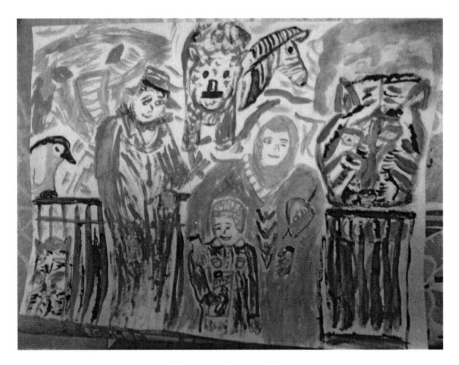

Painting, Bronx Zoo

When we arrive at the airport and get in the check-in line for Jet Blue, I am wheeling a little suitcase that has in it my computer, a sweater, my Kindle, and a few things too precious to check, such as my various pills and my camera. I also have a small plastic container of canned peaches, a food I can always eat. I know my carry-on allowance of liquid must be three ounces or less, unless (as the rules say) it's a container of breast milk for my baby. I don't know what my peaches weigh, but there are only three little slices in the container.

I put my suitcase on the conveyor belt along with my shoes, my laptop in a plastic tray, my jacket, and my purse, but I am stopped just before I pass through the metal detector machine. The TSA agent says, "Take off your hat."

"I have cancer," I tell him. "I am on chemo. I am bald."

He looks doubtful, but I'm playing the cancer card now. What I do is lift up my pink cap and let him see the truth of the violence of cancer. He sees my bald head and is shocked. Anyone else want to see it? Want to see if I'm going to blow up the plane with my bald head?

He waves me through but on the other side I am asked by a female TSA agent to surrender my little container of sliced peaches. "This is more than three ounces."

"Please, I need it. I'm on chemo; it's the only thing I can eat."

"Then you have to eat it right now," the woman says.

"Okay, I will." And I make them all wait, all the people in line going on their trips and all the TSA agents and all the Jet Blue pilots and all the flight attendants in the world have to wait for me to take out my little plastic spoon and chew, piece by piece, the three slices of sweet canned peaches, the food I need to stay alive. The terrorist they should fear is not me. It is cancer.

TWENTY-FIVE
SPILT MILK

Our first grandson is now six feet tall, suddenly manly, with a deep voice and enormous hands and feet that he will continue to grow into. His Oma, the grandmother from Berlin, and I sit on the porch of the rented house in DC and concur that if we were teenage girls, we would fall in love with him. We laugh. We have this beautiful bond, this understanding.

We have another understanding: that although she is both an MD and a psychoanalyst, neither my medical condition nor my mental state will be the focus of this visit.

I am careful to wear my caps and scarves in the public rooms. No one but my two-year-old granddaughter makes note of this. She says, "Grandma, why are you wearing a hat in the house?"

"To keep my head warm."

The true thrill of this event is my being in a space where all three of my daughters and their children are. This is wholeness for me. This is ecstasy. Joe and I and our three girls (and among them their five children)—what else could we ask for? The children have fathers—yes, of course, and I appreciate their contributions—but as a friend (also a mother of a daughter with children) once wrote me, "The children are always diluted by the father."

Still, we will all be together for two weeks. One week before the Bar Mitzvah and one week after. The rented home we are in is owned by a woman who loves books. Bookcases overflow in every room. The beds and chairs are high quality, real art decorates the walls and shelves, the dinnerware is fine china, and the appliances are modern and easy to use.

I am guaranteed by all that there is no work for me here. Others will shop and cook and do dishes and I will sit with the smaller children and tell them stories. Our first three grandchildren were boys—each one a delight and an education to a grandmother who had three girls—but now there are two granddaughters in the mix, and I am madly in love with these children.

Thank heaven, indeed, for little girls, with their apple cheeks, their joyful wild laughter, their streaming blonde hair (as they run through the house after each other), their (as it happens) blue eyes full of mischief. I want to touch them and kiss them. It's as if I am in love again. I think of them when they are not with me. I long for them. I want to see and hold them. Is such beauty the slyest trick of nature? Every baby is a seduction. Every baby invites lifelong bondage, service, adoration.

The boys, who are older—thirteen, eleven, six—play outside with manly things, baseball bats and balls (of course, balls). They use the bats as fencing swords. But the girls hang out with me. On my laptop computer I have years of photos of them and I show them their faces as babies, as little girls chasing butterflies in our backyard, swimming in our pool wearing their Floaties, eating buckets of chocolate ice cream in our kitchen. They cling to me, holding to either side of the chair where I sit at the desk in my rented bedroom and watching their own brief history unfold on the screen.

I entertain them with a YouTube video called "Cows, Cows, Cows," where the cows bounce and morph (to weird music) into tree cows, spider cows, bouncing cows, triple-headed cows, giraffe cows, wire cows. "Silly," says my littlest girl. "Funny," says the next oldest. I am in heaven here, and I get to kiss them so many times they begin to laugh and run away so I can run and catch them. (I can run! I am healthy! I am strong! They nourish me back to health.)

Family. This is the gift of the highest order. My daughters, separated by time and distance, living far from each other for years, catch up, talk for hours over coffee, or late at night over raspberry tea. They can't quite know my pride in them. That they are the monuments of my love and devotion and care ... and when I look at them now, I see how competent and wise and beautiful they are.

My cup runneth over with love.

In the two weeks we are in DC with the Berlin grandparents, there's a great flurry of activities. One night we go to the Filene Center at Wolf Trap National Park for the Performing Arts to see *Guys and Dolls*. A great rainstorm occurs during the performance. Fierce winds sweep the outdoor seats (under a protective roof covering) while the stars on stage sing "A Bushel and a Peck," a song full of love and hugs.

Love and lightning and wind and water—all the forces of life rage around us. The children huddle under their coats. The smallest grandchild still has her "blankie" and her pacifier to keep her safe. We are all in one row, close to the stage, again, all of us connected by blood, by choice, by love. How I love them all, a bushel and a peck.

After the show, those staying at my daughter's home say goodnight to us. We who are staying in the rented house drive home. The two sets of grandparents, my daughter Becky and her son Jacob, hang around to play Scrabble at the dining room table. We can hardly believe our luck—no one has school, no one has work, no one has bills to pay, my grandson's Bar Mitzvah is coming up on Saturday (tonight he will practice reading in Hebrew his Torah portion again) and after the great event, there will be a party here at this house to celebrate his becoming a man.

We drink from the bottle of wine Opa has in the refrigerator. We share some M&M's—not much plant-based food here—and we tell jokes. Tonight we have abandoned all worries, fears, anxieties, frustrations. As in the guided meditation tape, they are all flowing out of the bottoms of our feet with the muddy waters that poison us.

Just as we conclude it might be getting on to bedtime, there is a loud crash from the kitchen. Trouble! What could it be?

We discover that Becky's son, my grandson Jacob, has had a mishap with a dozen eggs. We are all in such a good mood that we admire his imagination as he makes a game of clean-up the kitchen floor. His goal is first to crush all the egg shells in his hands and listen to their satisfying crunch.

Joe comes over and puts his arm around me. It's clear we don't cry over spilt milk these days.

TWENTY-SIX
TODAY HE IS A MAN—THE BAR MITZVAH

THIS IS THE MORNING I COME face to face with God. I prepare for this by laying out my fancy clothes, by taking a shower. I no longer have the pleasure of washing my hair. What hair? Nor are there curls to blow this way and that with the dryer, to fluff up or scrunch tight. What curls? In my youth I used to have long hair. Joe often told me how much he loved my long hair.

Where these days are my feminine wiles? I see, as I shower, that I do have my breasts, my precious breasts, one and three-quarter breasts, not quite the full measure, but still there they are, on my body. They are still quite beautiful and I am alive.

My daughters each have breasts, and now, because of me, they have a *first degree* relative with breast cancer. My granddaughters will have breasts, and they now have a grandmother who has breast cancer. Five sets of breasts connected to me genetically. My children and grandchildren, like me, are mortal. Our little boys and girls who are with us so adorably, so full of life, so full of their unfolding futures, will one day, like me, die.

I can't picture this certainty without a gasp in my throat. But this is no way to prepare for a party! Give it up, Merrill! Do something useful. Go for a walk.

And why not take a walk in my party clothes? My Bar Mitzvah outfit is already on the bed. We are to leave for the synagogue in an hour, so let's put it on. Satiny slacks with a gauzy overlay, an embossed black and green top, sling-back black sandals, and of course my head covering, the cap, and over it a sparkling scarf shot with golden threads.

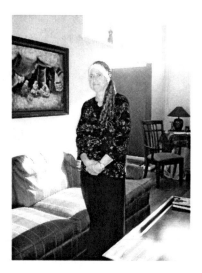

Merrill in party clothes and scarf

I tell no one I'm leaving. Joe and the Berlin grandparents are engaged in discussion in the kitchen. I take the house key from the hook in the hall and I'm on my way. What a fine morning to take a walk! Here in the East, the air is different. The rain cleanses the countryside nearly every day, the woods are deep and rich in tones of green and brown, and the sky is elegant with new bands of clouds moving in.

I appreciate every house on the block. I turn a corner: new houses, a new view, a long street ahead of me. Another corner, but now, where am I exactly? I read the street signs but they don't seem familiar. I think I have turned two corners or was it three, but am I walking a square route? How do I get back to the rented house? Do I even know the address there? Or the phone number? But I have no phone with me, in any case.

The wind is blowing a bit harder and my elegant gauzy pants begin to flap as I try to get back to the rented house where I live on a street whose name I don't even recall. My grandson will be Bar Mitzvahed this morning without me, and I will be alone and lost on these windy streets.

Suddenly I hear footsteps behind me. I glance over my shoulder and an astonishing vision confronts me. It's Joe! My husband Joe. He's come to find me. He's found me! I turn and run to him, my arms outstretched. Like a scene in a romantic movie, we fly in slow motion toward each other (slow motion because these sandals do not fit so well), and we hug with a force I don't remember since the days of our honeymoon.

I want a honeymoon again. I want those days in a Miami Beach Hotel. My honeymoon in a hotel on the edge of the Atlantic Ocean, where I first learned to love orange marmalade on my toast. My honeymoon that forever after caused me, by eating orange marmalade at breakfast, to want to have sex by dinnertime.

"When I didn't find you in the house, I had to come looking for you," Joe says.

"Of course you did." His face is so gorgeous, his jaw so square. My beloved.

And then my ankle turns in a small ditch between sidewalk and lawn, my heel slips out of its sling-back, and I fall hard on my knee. *Oh no!*

Is there is no end to trouble in life? Joe helps me up; it is quite a struggle. Holding onto him, I limp back to the house, which turns out to be blocks away. My knee hurts. I may need a knee replacement. I lie down on the bed to rest, rumpling my party clothes. Ahead of me is the encounter with God in the *shul*.

Then we are off, in several cars, to the synagogue. As we are about to file into the house of worship, I wonder at my discomfort. As a child, I would often go on Jewish holidays with my father and my aunt to the Ave N shul in Brooklyn—but to me it was a time to play outside with children from my neighborhood. My mother had no use for praying, for religious requirements, for the dietary commandments.

Yet here, about to take place, is the great and serious ritual for my grandson, one that has required years of Hebrew school, years of attendance at services, and years of contemplating the God of the Old Testament (a God who in my religion class at college struck me as vengeful, cruel, hot-tempered, self-centered, and narcissistic—the kind of man I would never marry, much less bow down to and worship).

Joe and I are going to be called up to the bima to stand beside our grandson as he reads his Torah portion. We already knew this and were given the prayer to say when called to stand beside him:

> Blessed are You, Lord our God, King of the Universe, who chose us from all the people and gave to us his Torah of truth and set everlasting life in our midst. Blessed are You, Lord, giver of the Torah.

The synagogue is a beautiful building. How I long to take photos of this event, but no cameras are allowed. A newsletter I had picked up in the lobby says, "G-d is taking all calls today … cell phones are not needed! Cell phones and pagers are prohibited in the synagogue building and on synagogue grounds on holidays and Shabbat."

But look, there is my grandson, on the bima, standing with the rabbi, standing above the great open Torah, standing with the *yad,* the silver pointer, in his hand. Joe and I are invited to say our prayer. The Berlin grandparents do likewise.

My grandson begins to read his Haftarah portion—my first grandson, the tiny boy I held on my lap and felt his surging, forceful energy of life.

How handsome, how tall he is. How beautifully the white prayer tallis with its fringes rests on his broad shoulders. And his voice … a man's voice that replaced the boy's voice magically just weeks before. He has learned the tongue of his forefathers; he is carrying on the great traditions of three thousand years. I should have given my daughters Hebrew educations. On my program I see a summary, written by my grandson, of today's Haftarah portion:

God speaks of the aid he has given the Israelites and the aid he will give them in the future. God says he will sustain them, make them flourish, and help them defeat enemies (and moreover, commands them to). God reminds the Jewish people of the hardships they have endured, and how he has helped them through those hardships. God warns the Israelites to stay loyal and not turn to idolatry or there will be dire consequences.

God tells the nation of Israel that it is not forgotten. God promises that the Israelites will have God's protection and that they will return to Zion, their homeland. They will be powerful and other nations will bow down before them. Later in the passage, God, speaking through the prophet Isaiah, scolds the people of Israel for being sinful and neglectful, reprehending them for deserting God.

Well, this is probably the vocabulary that turned me off decades ago: warnings, dire consequences, defeating enemies, commands, bowing down, scolding, being sinful and neglectful, reprehending.

Still, we are here in this awesome flow of history and mystery. It's best to surrender to it now and question it later. How proud we all are, to have come alive to this moment.

Outside, through the windows of the shul, the sky darkens. Thunder suddenly rattles the windows. The beating of rain begins to chatter against the sides of the building. Sizzles of lightning illuminate the room. God seems to want to make a loud and blazing commentary to accompany the chanting of the sacred words of the Torah.

The lights go out. We are all struck silent for a minute, for two minutes. But then, a faltering dimming blink and the lights come on again. What great relief we feel. God has saved us. He has protected us and we will return to Zion. My grandson has said his piece without error; he has come through this daunting ritual with excellence. He is smiling. We are all smiling, full of pride. The program continues, the rabbi says some words of congratulations.

The Sisterhood presents my grandson with an engraved Kiddush cup.

At the Kiddush event following, we all share food and wine. Some friends present gifts to the young man by way of small white envelopes. No fountain pens are offered, so far as I can tell. The children from the playroom have joined us. I see the rabbi pass by my grandson's little sister. He pauses to caress gently the top of her head. She looks up, sees him, and smiles so sweetly, I am touched almost to tears. She feels he is part of her family. She too, in eight years, will take her place on the bima and enter Jewish womanhood.

Much later, during the party at the rented house, when all my grandson's parents' friends and their children have joined us and we are busy talking and eating and celebrating, I go out on the upper back deck of the house and stand in awe of this world full of love, and in awe of the enormous pine tree in the yard. And in awe that I still have my life ahead of me, God willing.

TWENTY-SEVEN
AND THEN THE EARTH MOVED

THE DAY AFTER THE BAR MITZVAH there are a thousand pita breads left upon the table, there are four trays of an eggplant dish, three of Basmati rice, two of falafel balls, one tray of hummus and one of a delicious tahini sauce made with crushed sesame seeds, garlic and parsley. There is also a big round bowl of baba ganoush (what an amazing word!). Several cakes and pies are in the refrigerator. We have enough food to feed us for a month.

All the relatives convene in the rented house. The children find dozens of games in the playroom—one of which contains a thousand tiny colored-plastic circles and squares. Soon these are distributed throughout the house.

The youngest children also want to see again the YouTube video of "Cows, Cows, Cows" and stand transfixed before the computer in my bedroom watching the cows bounce like balls, grow like trees, turn into spiders, morph into giraffe cows, three-headed cows. The five children have bonded as if Super Glue has coated their spirits and knitted them into one organism. Though they live far from one another, in groups of two, two and one, they are like the points of a singular star: they glow and gleam with light and energy. How they laugh and roll on the floor and hide and trick one another! How the two eldest boys fence with plastic baseball bats, how the youngest boy and the two little girls run about in the yard, each with a pastel colored butterfly net!

I think if I should die here, watching them play, I would die happy.

How will we ever part from one another? How will we leave this harmonious camp and travel back to our specific lives—and what were they again? The two Berlin grandparents will go back to their country and their language. They will vanish into another world. My daughters will return to their homes, their jobs, their lives that I know only a little about, only what they wish to tell me. And I will go back home and into the jaws of cancer treatment. My first radiation session begins on September 1st ... I have marked the calendar.

TWO DAYS LATER JOE AND I are at our daughter's home with our grandson and his little sister; their parents have gone out with the others, gone out to lunch, gone shopping, but we four are sitting quietly in the compact, six-level townhouse. I am reading a book on the living room couch. My grandson is upstairs in his room with the door closed. His little sister and Joe are downstairs in the den playing with dinosaurs.

I hear a tremendous vibration. The walls are shimmering; the lamps are quivering. The earth moves, shifts—for a second it seems the walls threaten to fall in on me. Earthquake? We have them often in California, but what is happening here, now? An explosion? A bomb!

The earth is still moving. I leap up. "Joe! Where are you?"

There are footsteps thundering down the stairs and others coming up the stairs. Joe is carrying our granddaughter. We rush outside and stand, breathless, in the street. My grandson reaches for his little sister and holds her tight in his arms. She clutches him, her face pale. We stand in the hot summer afternoon on the grassy slope in front of the house. Others on the street have also come outside, baffled and alarmed.

I tell my grandson to run in and get the cordless phone. He does. In half a second he is in and out, and hands it to me. I call my sister in California. "Bobbie, turn on the TV. Tell us what happened out here."

In a minute we know: a 5.8 earthquake has struck in DC.

Amazement upon amazement. Is it God sending a message? First, thunder, lightning, rain, and now an *earthquake?* We four stand in the street, grateful to be together and safe. But where are the others? Are they safe?

It is at least an hour before we dare to go back into the house. By then, our daughter has been able to call to ask if we are okay and to tell us they are also safe. An earthquake in this part of the world is nearly a miracle. My grandson goes back to his room. Joe and our granddaughter go back down to the den to play with dinosaurs. As for me, I am thinking about going home in a few days to confront the powers of the linear accelerator.

The next day we learn of another possible catastrophe coming our way: Hurricane Irene is forming and is on its way to ravage the East Coast. It will strike the day before we and the Berlin grandparents are supposed to fly to our respective homes.

Joe and I have a disagreement. I want to fly out before the hurricane closes all the airports. I went to fly home to begin radiation treatments. Joe has been enlivened by all the adventures and dangers we have encountered here—he hasn't seen a hurricane since we both lived in Miami Beach in our teen years. He wants to stay for the hurricane. He wants to be here with our kids to protect them. He wants to help them stock up on food, batteries, a hand-held can opener, cans of tuna fish, water. I assure him they have the know-how to do this for themselves. But in some way, we all want to stay; we all want to huddle together with the ones we love. We want to face the elements as a band of warriors. We don't want to abandon our children—make our own escape and leave them to their fates.

But logic prevails. The German grandparents are on the phone to change their tickets to Berlin. They likewise are torn, but rational. We all need to get home while the planes are flying. We have that other life out there ... our responsibilities, our bill-paying, our medical appointments. Our children will be fine in a mere hurricane—they are not at the water's edge; they are in a strong brick townhouse lodged between two others. They are not near a river that will flood or an ocean that will rise. No tsunami is predicted.

Oma and Opa and Joe and I confer. We call our airlines. The lines are busy, busy, people are changing their air reservations. But there won't be a charge for these changes. If there are seats going where we have to go, we can get them.

Jet Blue finds seats for us on a flight to California—not next to each other, but separated. However, their representative assures us that kind passengers, seeing us old married people needing to hold hands during periods of turbulence, will move around, change seats, and let us sit together. Will the TSA agent make me take off my cap? Will they confiscate my little container of baba ganoush?

We have to hurry to pack up our things a day early. We have to say our goodbyes. The idyll has to end sooner or later. We promise one another we will all reconvene, at the very least, for our granddaughter's Bat Mitzvah. Or for our grandson's wedding. But sooner than that, we hope. Let us live and be well, we old grandparents admonish one another. We know exactly how old we are. There are no guarantees. Our youngest daughter and her family will fly out on one airline, Becky and Jacob on another. The pain of all this separation is almost too much for me. Hurricanes, earthquakes, airplanes, danger—and all of us marching into the wind without the others. As for me, I will be going home to face cancer. Back to the hunt and the eradication of the killer cells hiding in me, but where? Heaven knows.

TWENTY-EIGHT
A RIDE IN THE LINEAR ACCELERATOR

The walls of the hallway leading to the LINAC room are lined with lead.

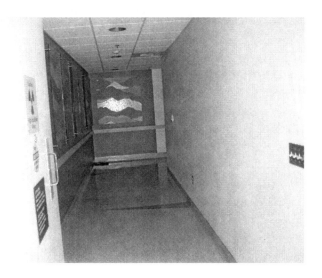

Hallway to LINAC

Once I begin the journey down this corridor, I am on my way to a new reality.

When I register for my appointment, the receptionist gives me a little palm-sized disk, exactly like the kind we have been given at the Romano's Macaroni Grill. When there is a table ready for us, the disk buzzes and a series of bright lights flicker on and off. Here, in the radiation center, the flashing buzzing disk is my signal to enter the hallway, begin my journey, and on the way, get two warm cotton blankets from a specialized oven and in a dressing room, put on my hospital gown:

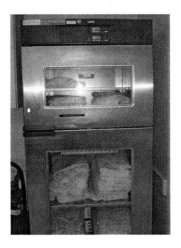

Blanket warmer radiation department

Then I enter the room with the monolith:

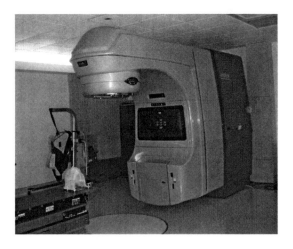

Monolith LINAC

I am positioned inside it:

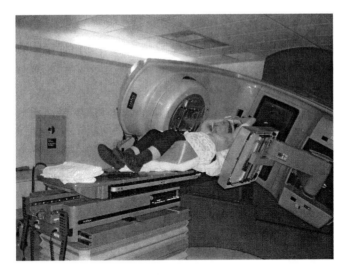

Merrill in LINAC

Simple as that. The techs line me up under green beams of light. They pull me this way and that ("Don't try to help us," they say), and when they are certain I am positioned properly, they run off down that hallway while a great thick door closes me inside the room. From a control area, far away, they push the button and the burning beams enter my body. A red light flashes, a loud clacking noise beeps continuously as I lie there, willing but baffled, feeling nothing but knowing something enormous is taking place. I count thirty-three clacking beeps. What else have I to do?

The red light goes off. I can see the leaden door, like a prehistoric animal roused from the sleep of a century, slowly move to an open position.

The two pretty techs come in and say "All done." They help me sit up, they unfurl my arms from the uncomfortable position behind my head, they tell me to dress and they remind me: "Remember to rub aloe vera gel on your breast now, during the day and at bedtime."

WE HAVE AN ALOE VERA PLANT in front of the house. Its leaves are as spiky as a cactus plant. I can't begin to equate the ooze from its spikes as a balm for my burns. Instead, in the clinic pharmacy, I buy a bottle of Fruit of the Earth Aloe Gel—"Totally Pure," and I return to the dressing room to rub some on my breast. There are dire warnings about radiation—burns and blisters possible on my skin, extreme fatigue that will increase with the days of treatment. Dr. Goy has given me a prescription for a cortisone cream that will relieve the itching of my burned flesh.

My flesh has already taken a beating. The chemo and the daily baby aspirin I take have turned my skin from a protective covering to a covering that needs protection. Any tiny bump of my hand—against the side of a door, the inside of the pantry cabinet, the top of my underwear drawer—will scrape away inches of skin. I bleed. My hands turn into a polka-dot pattern of black and purple scars and bruises.

These are the hands of a very old woman. These images are the forerunners of death. But let us not go there, Merrill. This Merrill has to be hit on the head with a lead pipe to shut off those tapes of gloom. Go for a walk, Merrill.

So Joe and I go to lunch in Ontario after my treatment. We find an inviting coffee shop a few blocks away. We order giant breakfasts, eggs and bacon and pancakes and home fried potatoes. I pour (fake) maple syrup over my entire plate. Though I haven't ordered toast, there are free tiny boxes of jelly in a tray on the table. I put six of them containing orange marmalade into my purse. Orange marmalade, my aphrodisiac potion. I get up and walk to the next (empty) booth and I steal the orange marmalade boxes from their holder. I would go even farther to another booth, but Joe stops me. "Sit down and eat."

He knows I have criminal tendencies like this. I attribute them to the fact that my father was an antique dealer (a secondhand junk dealer), and that every object we ever had in our Brooklyn house had been used first by someone else who either died or discarded it. But perhaps there's something deeper behind it: I need more than I have. I need enough. I need enough to feel safe, enough of everything, enough jelly. I really need my children to be close to me. I need safety and softness. I have a down comforter on my already soft memory-foam bed. I have a puffy, down-filled jacket. I like warm things and soft things and safe things.

I dreamed last night that I was walking on the beach and saw on a boardwalk bench a pink knitted baby blanket. In the dream, I pick it up to take it home. I want to give it to my granddaughter, whose own baby blanket is in shreds. But once I get home and unfold the blanket, I see it is a beautiful, hand-embroidered Indian shawl with individually sewn teardrop pearls hanging from its edges. Not only that, but a sheet of paper falls from it, and on it is written the list of shawls that the Indian woman has made and sold. Each one costs $385 dollars. This is *her* list.

What shall I do? I wrap the pink beaded shawl around my neck. It unfolds down to the floor, a beautiful, elegant, magnificent evening wrap. I will never go anywhere I could wear such a wrap. It is for a young and beautiful woman. And how will I explain it to Joe? He will be angry with me for taking it in the first place. It is not mine!

And where shall I hide it from him? It is all a tangle of pain and grief and guilt and theft.

But something has been taken from me! There is a hole in me where my breast was once whole. Something deadly has been scooped out of me. I need something to fill it. I need marmalade and safety. I need to be the young woman who can dance the night away in that shimmering pink-beaded Indian shawl.

After lunch, Joe and I go to see one of the cow farms in Ontario.

How peaceful it looks. Acres of green grass—and there are the cows, rows upon rows of them. These cows in Ontario are trusting, lined up at their food bins. They have no clue they are destined for the butcher block. Meat! Most of my friends in the cancer support group have given up eating meat.

I am hungry, suddenly. I didn't eat any of the eggs, bacon, or pancakes. I can't swallow food like that. I want something soft and sweet.

"Joe, find me a McDonald's. I want a McCafé Mocha with ice cream, coffee, chocolate, and whipped cream."

"Didn't we just have lunch a few minutes ago?"

But he sees by my face that there's no rational person in the mind behind it. We drive almost all the way home, and Joe takes me to the McDonald's a few blocks from our house, the one where we used to take our children, where we all used to order Big Macs and french fries and a ton of ketchup.

TWENTY-NINE
MISCALCULATION AT THE INFUSION CENTER

THE MONTH OF RADIATION DOESN'T EXCUSE me from my chemo infusions—but there is good news, says Dr. Bracamonte. The new infusion center has just opened, a gorgeous space at the entrance to the hospital. We will no longer have to travel to the third floor, along sinuous hallways, to that crowded—overcrowded—space where the infusion chairs are close together, where the wooden handles used to recline the chairs are often stuck and don't work.

Best of all, Dr. B says, is the wonderful view of the spacious pond and a glimmering fountain.

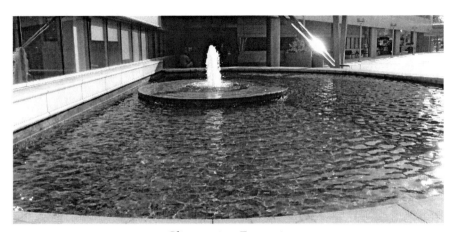

Glimmering Fountain

But there has been a miscalculation. All the chairs in the infusion room have their backs to the fountain. The electric plugs are in the wall, and the chairs face away from the windows. Furthermore, now that the chairs are so far apart and the cubicles separated by curtains, there is no way to visit with fellow cancer friends, exchange news, encouragement, and food.

Even more disturbing is that every infusion chair now has its own TV. This means that every few feet someone is listening to a loud TV show. The racket is incredible.

Try to read? Impossible. Try to listen to music? Impossible. On one side of my chair, a shoot-'em-up Western is playing, and on the other is a screaming game show. Peace is gone. My view is of the other inside wall.

My dear nurse Cristina is apologetic. She finds the racket awful, too.

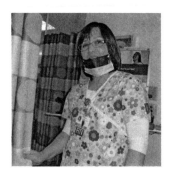

Chemo nurse Cristina Mateo

Still, she is my comfort every time I arrive for an infusion. Her magical technique of finding one of my veins still available is a blessing. Chemo has damaged my veins and made them so delicate that they are in danger of blowing out when a needle is inserted. Dr. B suggests I could have an infusion port. However, the infusion port must be installed surgically—a device that is implanted in my chest and from which a catheter is threaded to my heart. This would allow infusions to be done more easily, without the pain of a needle-stick, and available quickly in an emergency.

But another surgery? And then, even after chemo is finished, it is advised that one leave the port in place "in case." The "in case" means in case cancer comes back. And if it's left in place, it must be flushed with saline solution every month or two to keep it open and available. That means coming back to the infusion center forever, or so it seems to me. I would rather suffer the sticks of the needles. Especially with Cristina's gentle and careful sensing of where an open vein can be found.

Still, the noise unsettles me. Game shows and news and old movies! (There is a censor in these TVs—no R-rated movies, no violent police shows.) I don't want to be forced to listen to this noise. Before this great new infusion center opened, while still in the old one, I would bring my Kindle, a gift to me from my youngest daughter, and read to my heart's content. I am unable now to read even my own manuscript, which I downloaded as a document.

In every waiting room at this medical facility there has always been a TV—one can't escape them. They are there to distract, to help one escape from the worry of a medical visit. But while one is taking chemo into her veins, while one is trying to heal, while one is considering guided meditation in the infusion chair, when one wants music and poetry, one gets inescapable, unbearable, competing TV shows blaring at full volume.

"I won't go back," I tell Joe. "I'll quit having chemo."

"Write a letter," Joe tells me. "Write a magic letter. You know what you can do with a letter."

"I'll write a letter to the head of the Oncology Department," I agree.

I write an email, not a letter, and two days later I have a reply from the administrative director of the Oncology Department. He agrees that the noise problem has to be addressed. He is going to order earphones that patients can use. Furthermore, until the earphones arrive, he will have a volume control installed in each TV to keep the noise level down.

The power of the pen is mighty, indeed. Thank heaven.

THIRTY
MEALS ON WHEELS! $2 SENIOR LUNCH!

W E ARE IN DESPERATE STRAITS. THE daily sixty-mile round trip for my radiation treatments has worn us out. We come right home, I rub aloe vera on my breast, and I go to bed and nap. No one shops. No one cooks. No one buys Chinese egg drop soup or canned peaches. Not an egg is in the refrigerator. Not a single noodle.

A friend says we need Meals on Wheels. Well, of course we don't. That's for old, sick people, isn't it? I call their number and a woman comes to our house to interview us. Well, we are old and sick. We qualify. A delivery will take place once a week, on Tuesday morning. Seven frozen meals will be delivered for me, seven for Joe: seven slices of wheat bread each, seven pieces of fruit each, and seven little containers of milk for each of us.

To me this sounds like heaven. I can't go on not eating, losing weight. Joe thinks this is all unnecessary, but I have to face the truth: if I leave it to him to feed me, I will starve.

We make room in the freezer for the first delivery, which means throwing out all the long forgotten and unrecognizable items covered with frost. A truck pulls up on the next Tuesday, and a woman carries an insulated case into our kitchen. She personally has to see that there's room in the freezer; she will personally put the frozen meals into it. We have a problem though—we will be away for my radiation treatments for all the following Tuesdays of the month.

Marcie, the delivery person, is stumped; she's not allowed to leave the food at the door or with a neighbor. What if we hide a key? Can she put the food in our freezer? She isn't really supposed to do that either, but under these special circumstances, if we all keep it a secret, she'd be happy to let herself in and deliver the food.

The first night we examine some of our choices:

Fish with Hollandaise Sauce. That doesn't sound bad.

Then there's Meatballs & Gravy. Not so bad either.

We are set for at least a month. We are grateful. A little envelope comes with the delivery. We may make a donation or not; it's purely a suggestion.

This is a life-saver, but it's not high cuisine. These meals satisfy the need for dinner, but what about lunch? We no longer want to go to a coffee shop and order some huge meal after my treatment. Radiation does make me tired. I want to get home.

Then, driving home from radiation treatment one day, I see a sign at the community center a block from our house. "Senior Lunch $2"—ALL SENIORS WELCOME.

"Let's try that," I say. Joe is dubious, but I'm adamant. The next day we walk the short block to the park. We live in a wonderful place, nestled (as they say) in the shadows of the foothills of the San Gabriel Mountains. Just a block from our house is the community recreation center, the community swimming pool, and the city's small and beautiful Pioneer Cemetery.

Tables for the seniors are already set with plastic utensils. We are welcomed, we sign in, and we each place two dollars in a little brown envelope and put the envelopes in a box. There is a menu for the week posted. I begin to feel as if I could start eating again. Lunch here, dinner at home. The terrible riddle of where to find food is being solved.

This lunch is lovely—fresh vegetable soup (I can eat soup!), teriyaki chicken and rice, salad, and peach cobbler, all served on a Styrofoam tray. We talk to the other elders at the table—they have their reasons for being here. One woman in her nineties comes with her aide. A Chinese couple comes because "My wife doesn't like to cook." Another man comes because he is blind; a friend guides him. We have just entered a new phase of life, as bona fide old folks. If we want to come every day, we have to sign up for a week at a time.

I don't eat much, but I eat something. Joe eats everything. On Fridays, we learn, the chef from a local retirement home comes with special baked goods for everyone—cupcakes, apple pie, beautifully decorated cookies. Of course this is an advertising event, but it's appreciated. Who knows? We may all need a retirement home not long from now.

We go for lunch every day. The walk to the park does us good. We take nothing with us but two dollars each. The air is fresh, and the mountains are brilliant with the green of pine trees. These mountains have burned in the past, in the hot dry days of summer, but now they are burgeoning again.

I am getting through radiation treatments. I am feeling hopeful. There is a box on the desk at the radiation center where women beginning to get their hair back can leave their caps and scarves for those who need them. My entire treatment takes about ten minutes. My skin is not yet burning. My skin is not yet itching. The blisters in my mouth have healed. And is it possible? My hair is beginning to grow back.

Each night now, when Joe knows it's time for me to apply the aloe vera gel, he asks, "Would you like me to do it for you?" He warms the gel in his hand and then he gently applies it to my breast. He is very careful. He is very loving. How I love him.

Toward the end of the month of treatment, I get my "boost"— the extra radiation to the scar area. My breast is a little sunburned, perhaps a little smaller now, as the radiation shrinks the skin. The tattoo is still visible. It's my souvenir.

And on the last day I get yet another souvenir—my certificate of completion.

When we get home on this day, we go down to the Senior Lunch. I am full of happiness and joy. I have lived through radiation. I tell the woman at the lunch sign-in desk that I've finished my treatment. Then I tell her how good the food is here, and how much better it is than Meals on Wheels.

Her face darkens. "You're getting Meals on Wheels?"

"Yes, I am."

"Well, you can't have lunch here and get meals delivered, too. It's illegal! I'm going to have to report you."

"Report me?"

"You can't double-dip!" she admonishes me.

And we're cancelled from Meals on Wheels. We cancel ourselves from the Senior Lunch. I am getting better. We don't need these services anymore. We will make our own meals. We are able now to fend for ourselves.

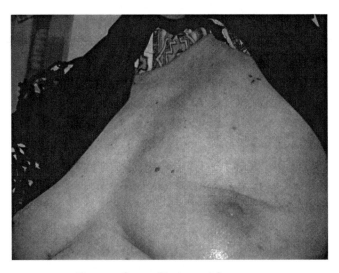

Breast after radiation with tattoo

THIRTY-ONE
GENETIC COUNSELING, THE DEVIL-CHASER

THREE WOMEN IN MY CANCER GROUP have the Braca gene mutation.

Two of them have ovarian cancer. One has been identified as having the mutation but has not decided what steps to take. Women who have this mutation have a much higher risk for breast and other cancers. More than 85 percent will one day develop breast cancer.

All three of them know young women who, each having been identified with the mutation, elected because the risk is so high to have their breasts, ovaries, and uteruses removed.

I've told those in my group that I am Jewish. That my ancestors were from Eastern Europe, that my grandmother came alone to this country at the age of seventeen to find her fortune. By leaving Poland before Hitler took it over, she saved her own life and of course the lives of my mother and her sisters, and therefore also my life and those of my sister, my children, and their children.

The fact is that women of Ashkenazi Jewish descent are at the highest risk for mutated Braca genes. If I have the gene mutation, my daughters will be at risk.

Becky comes with me to an appointment with a genetic counselor. The counselor takes a detailed history of the cancers in my family. Do I really know who had cancer? My father's mother died of a "stone in the stomach." My own father died of leukemia, which whisked him from health to death in three months. How I wish he had kept the devil-chaser and not given it to me. Maybe it would have saved him. What a strange, antique artifact it is, designed to chase away evil. Its devil face, wearing a hat of cymbals, is perched on a long wooden stick with a spring at the bottom so it can be banged up and down. The racket chases away those evil spirits that wish to do us harm.

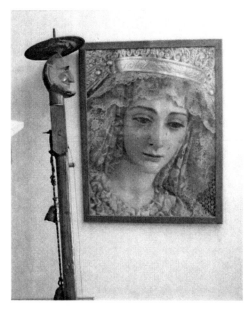

Devil-chaser and Madonna of Tears

I keep it in my office next to a Madonna of Tears, an image I found in a thrift shop. Her face seems beautiful and touching to me. A devil-chaser, the image of the Mother of God, my four-leaf clover necklace … who can say what protects us, or what fools us into thinking we are protected?

I dutifully list the cancers I know of: my father's two sisters died of cancer, one of cervical cancer, one of laryngeal cancer. His uncles died of mysterious things—perhaps cancers, perhaps not. My mother, her sisters, and my grandmother all had devastating strokes, but not cancer. My mother's first cousin had breast cancer twice in her young years, and another first cousin was stricken with it at 103. She had two male first cousins who died of pancreatic cancer, of colon cancer.

Who doesn't have a family rife with cancer?

The chart the geneticist draws up looks like a puzzle.

She concludes that because none of my first-degree relatives died young of breast or ovarian cancer and because I got cancer when I was no longer young, it is unlikely that I carry the Braca mutation.

She denies me permission to have the blood test. Becky and I are worried. I am an Ashkenazi Jewish woman with breast cancer. If I have the gene, I should know.

My friends in the Cancer Support Community are outraged. My friend, who is eighty-three and Jewish and in the same medical system as I am in, got the test. "The squeaky wheel gets the oil," she insists. "Make a fuss. You're entitled."

"Do it for your daughters," my friend who carries the gene mutation advises me.

I think I should do it for my daughters. I wait some weeks. I wait some months. One day I stumble on a small article in the newspaper: Medicare now supports Braca gene testing for all Jewish women who have breast cancer.

I send an email to the geneticist. She meets with the head of her department, a MD *and* a geneticist, and they agree to let me have the test.

I have to have other blood work in any case, so the order is added to my lab list. I get my blood drawn by a lab tech who puts a hot compress on my right arm (left arm: no needles, no BP), and blood is drawn.

Two weeks later I get the news: no genetic abnormalities. I call my daughters, one by one. *Whew!* The devil-chaser worked.

THIRTY-TWO
BUYING CEMETERY REAL ESTATE

WE ARE GOING TO DIE. WE have managed in some fashion to ignore that fact for more than the fifty-some years of our marriage, but it's coming into sharper focus these days. Our parents have all died, all of our aunts and uncles have died, and some of our friends have died.

My Aunt Thelma, technically my mother's first cousin, is now 106. Her sister died at 103. The two women lived in Florida, in adjacent buildings, but hadn't talked to one another in forty years. Neither of them could remember why they had fought, but they knew they had. I still talk to my Aunt Thelma frequently; she remembers my mother in her girlhood, she remembers how handsome my father was, she knows family secrets, and she tells them to me. I once encouraged her to write the story of her life; she wrote it in longhand, and I made photocopies of it for all her nieces and nephews. She has no children.

She was once a secretary to a man who owned a cemetery; now she owns the cemetery. I don't know if she will be buried there. We haven't discussed her burial; it seems an awkward subject. "I know I have to die but I don't want to die," she said when last we spoke.

She took a fall and broke her hip and now she lives in her apartment on the Florida waterfront creek with three round-the-clock aides. But still she handles her investments, her menu for her meals. She still paints and plays the piano.

But who can bank on getting to 106?

Joe and I live one block from the Pioneer Cemetery. We have a view of it from our pool deck.

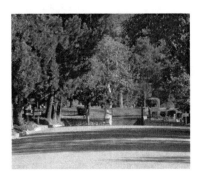

Cemetery from my Window

Every Fourth of July, the city parade passes by the cemetery, bands playing, the Search and Rescue Dogs marching by, the singular belly dancer who has been in the parade for the last thirty-five years twirling her veil (but wearing sneakers).

At the parade's end, the great fire trucks pass by the cemetery, their sirens roaring, their horns honking. Just as they pass the entrance to the cemetery in the blasting heat of summer, the firemen turn on their water hoses. The children wait for this moment, carrying their own water weapons to aim at the firemen.

I have to hide my camera at that moment or it will be soaked, but the water is sprayed far and wide—cool, and beautiful—clear into the cemetery. The first of the dead buried there in 1884 was a Civil War veteran. Following him to the burial grounds came the dead of the Spanish American War, World Wars One and Two, the Korean War, the Vietnam War. None yet, so far as I know, from the Iraq or Afghanistan wars. The dead, each July 4th, are sprinkled with this happy watery benediction, the grace of a free country falling on the tombstones and the crosses.

And there's the rub, for us. All those crosses. From our sleuthing, we discovered only two graves with Stars of David on them. There are also angels on the graves, American flags, dolls, a toy piano. Now and then we've seen a burial taking place—family members standing in the grass, a Scottish bagpipe player blowing mournful tunes over the graves.

I think we should be buried here, in this burial ground that is almost like our front yard, in the shadow of the grand mountain that stands majestic in the view from our kitchen window. It sends its breezes to our house; it glows golden as the sun hits its tip every morning. We've lived in its image for forty-five years. We came to this house as a young married couple with three small children and breathed the air here every day for 16,000 days. (I did the math.)

There's one small problem. We already own burial sites in Mt. Sinai, the Jewish cemetery where my mother and father are buried, where my aunt and uncle are buried. After my mother died, we bought these graves secondhand, from a man who was moving back to New York and planned to die there with his wife. These graves were a steal—not two steps from the curving road near the cemetery entrance but also under two canopied shade trees. These are prime sites. Dead Jews were overrunning the cemetery, which had begun expanding up into the hills, then into even higher and rockier hills. At present the earthmovers are digging gravesites that are almost inaccessible and yet are selling for more than twice what we paid.

I had recently inquired about the cost of burial there: to own the gravesites was barely the beginning. I had a list of what was required for us to be deposited in consecrated Jewish ground: "Basic services, $1350." "Transfer of remains, $375." (Wasn't that a basic service?) "Standard preparation: $450." (What was that?) "Embalming—$450." (We weren't interested in embalming.) "Use of funeral coach: $100." "Outer burial vault/grave liner: $550." "Cemetery charges, open/close: $800." Then there was the burial shroud, $150, newspaper notice, $100, Limousine, $700, Flowers, $400+, Rabbi Honorarium, $500+, and Memorial tablet, $2000+.

All these thousands, just for being deposited in consecrated Jewish earth? Right next door to the Jewish cemetery was the famous Forest Lawn, a Christian cemetery. Did God differentiate between Jewish soil and Christian soil?

Never mind. The Pioneer Cemetery has a small fee for burial, even smaller if you want a cremation plot, and smaller yet if you want to be buried in the Cremation Garden, a square of dirt that could contain thousands of cremains, the mere dust of the dead. Their names are engraved on a plaque on the wall.

Joe and I make a date to meet a representative who knows where new graves have been designated for sale. This cemetery has been full for years, but recently they added a grassy hillside of graves and chose a few paths that could now also be offered as graves.

Joe and I walk down the block to the cemetery. Half in a joking mood, he says he wants a statue of himself on a horse on his grave like the one he saw in Rome of Victor Emanuel, King of Italy. I say I want my writing name, Merrill Joan Gerber, not my married name, on my grave. I'd also like an image of a typewriter on mine and I think Joe should have a piano on his.

I remember the words on a gravestone I once saw in a Boston graveyard. I took the first line of it for the title of my first published book, *Stop Here, My Friend*.

> Stop Here, My Friend
> As You Pass By
> As You Are Now
> So Once Was I
> As I Am Now
> So You Will Be
> Prepare for Death
> And Follow Me!

All this presupposes the unbearable, that one day we will be separated from each other, one of us dead before the other, one of us still alive in the house down the street and the other dead and in ashes a block away in the Pioneer Cemetery.

Dead and cold. I think of my mother underground in her

bathrobe with little red sailboats on it, buried now sixteen years, her bathrobe housing a skeleton. "I want to be cremated," I tell Joe. "I want to vanish in a whoosh of flame. It's cleaner than rotting away."

"What if we're all called up in the Rapture, and you don't have your skeleton in which to be reconstituted?"

"I'll worry then."

Is this a joking matter? It's such a beautiful day. The cemetery is aglow with sunshine, with fresh flowers on some graves, and we can hear the cries of children playing in the playground down the hill.

We pick a likely tree to be buried under.

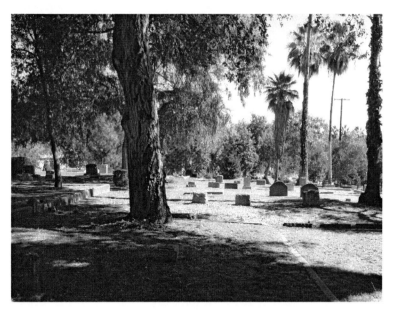

Our cemetery plots

Yes, there are two cremation graves available under that very tree, the woman who finds us there tells us. In fact, if we buy two cremation graves, we can actually have the cremains of four people in them. Room for more. Fun for the whole family!

We make a deal on the spot. She does the paperwork. We sign on the dotted line.

* * *

WALKING HOME, WE WONDER: WHAT HAVE we done? But I'm not unsettled by this move. I'm actually reassured. Buying our graves is no speedy invitation to our deaths. In fact, we've now pushed those events so far into the future, we can forget about them in the present.

THIRTY-THREE
A CROWN OF SNOW-WHITE HAIR

◦⟋◦

D R. B PROMISED ME IT WOULD happen. My hair would come back. And now it's coming back. Not so much, at first, but enough. A crown of snow-white hair.

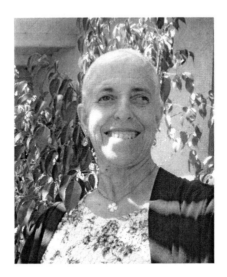

A crown of snow-white hair

Who is this white-haired woman? Well, she's my mother, of course. She's also my grandmother. When I was ten or eleven, in Brooklyn, I'd walk my grandmother from Ave O to Ave P, to the

Claridge Theater, where we'd buy tickets to the movies. As we paid for our tickets on Saturdays, we'd each get a free dish or a plate or a cup. If we came to the movies every week, in time we would have a whole set of new dishes.

My grandmother would give me money to buy Jujubes or Good & Plenty, and I'd go to the candy counter. On the way back, I'd count rows down the aisle until I saw the gleaming white hair of my grandmother. She had perfectly white, perfectly brilliant glowing white hair. She was snow on a mountaintop. She was a fluffy white bird. Homing in on her, I would never get lost.

So now I have become my grandmother. Become my mother, whose hair also turned white in her youth. Joe likes my white hair. It's "age appropriate," he says. I'm not sure what that means. That I look like an old lady, and I am an old lady?

But where are my curls? I always had curly hair. It was my birthright, my trademark. "Merrill's beautiful curly hair," my aunt, the hairdresser would say. "Just look at her. Who wouldn't die to have hair like that?"

Well, I nearly did die, and now I have hair like this, and I'm ever grateful. Away go all the caps and scarves—the wigs have long since been dumped in a box.

I test my new hair in the world; I now get without question a senior discount at the thrift shop. Now that I am shopping and cooking again, I sometimes ask the supermarket checker if someone can unload my basket for me. What's surprising is that the supermarket checkers are disappearing. Instead, in several stores where I shop, three little stations replace the checkout counter and each patron is advised to "self check out" his own food. This means lifting each item, locating the barcode on it, and scanning it across the glass strip below. Is someone spying above us? How can they trust us to scan every item? How do they know that when I press the "banana" button, and the screen asks "how many?" that I don't press 3 when I have 5? How do they know I don't scan one can of tuna fish, but push through two? This is very complicated. A voice will suddenly say "An unidentified item is on the scanner. Please remove it." Is it my purse that's unidentified? Is it the tissue that fell out of my pocket?

"Hello, can you help me?" I ask various people wearing green aprons. "I have no idea what I'm doing."

Not only do I have to self-check, I have to self-package. Some markets have banned the use of plastic grocery bags and post reminders at the entrance: "Don't forget your carry bags!" However, because I *have* forgotten them, and because my car is parked far back in the lot, I will just go in without my carry bags and buy paper bags for ten cents apiece.

It won't be long before we shoppers are meeting the trucks in the loading area and carrying in the food and stocking it ourselves on the shelves.

Today I am in a market where there is a real checker. She checks, she scans my card, she tells me the total, and she says, "Would you like to make a contribution to breast cancer?"

"I *have* it," I tell her. "I *have* breast cancer."

What does it mean, that I say that? That I don't think donations for breast cancer research are worthy? That after all these years of research, and after all my donations at the checkout, I got breast cancer anyway? Or am I just playing my cancer card?

I'm sorry to have blurted out to this checker the thought that lives inside me every minute of my life.

"Do you need help to your car?"

"No, I don't." I'm sorry I didn't say yes, because I do need help to my car. Can't she see by my white hair that I need help?

I push my cart, loaded with food now that we don't do the $2 Senior Lunch or Meals on Wheels. This is food that I will have to put away in the refrigerator, plan a meal around—cook the chicken, steam the rice, boil a vegetable, make a salad. I imagine the movements necessary for these actions—in speeded-up motion I see my hands flying like karate-chops—whack, spin, smash, slice, cut, stir, fry, bake, toast. I think of the days when my children were little: five meals to be made, three times a day. Six braids on three little girls to be braided every day. An entire house to manage, organize, clean, wipe, vacuum.

One day, a day very like this one, when the girls were little and I had been out shopping for food, I came home and found the front door partly open. *Crooks! A break-in!* I dared not go inside. I went to my neighbor's house and called the police.

In a minute the squad car pulled up in front of my house.

"You found the door open?" the policeman asked.

"Yes."

I followed him to the front door, watched him kick open the door, watched him place his hand on the gun in his holster. I stood behind him as he stared into our living room. There on the floor was a tangle of clothing, toys tossed here and there, pajamas, hairbrushes, hair ribbons, books, a few pots, shoes.

"Someone has been ransacking your house, ma'am," the officer said.

"Oh, no," I assured him. "That's how it looks every morning by the time I get the girls off to school."

In the end, the policeman found no burglars. He concluded the door had swung open by itself, not having been properly closed. I thanked him for his help.

Today, as I carry groceries into the house, bag by bag, food for just the two of us, I see the living room is as neat and empty as if two ghosts lived here. Joe and I are the ghosts. We are the old folks with white hair. Our staying time in this house is coming to an end. When? No one knows. That's why I shop. That's why I keep the wheels turning—because we are alive. I will cook that chicken. I will make a glorious dinner for us. I will light candles at the table. We are here to stay for a good long while.

THIRTY-FOUR
CANNABIS AND CUPCAKES

❧

Finally comes the day of the end of formal treatment. Of course, Dr. B will want to see me every three months for five years; she will want blood work done before every visit, measuring what blood can measure, including the two breast cancer numbers. The CEA should be below 5. Once it was up to 6 and she was concerned: have you been near a forest fire? Have you been near people who are smoking? Smoke can raise those numbers.

But no, I had been nowhere smoky, unless you count the toast burning one morning. But the test three months later revealed the CEA number had dropped to 4.2.

"These numbers vary. You can't jump to conclusions. You wait to see the trend. We look for trends."

Though my chemo is coming to an end, my toes, damaged by peripheral neuropathy, are still numb, lumpy, cold. They always feel peculiar. I will never have my old toes back, and who knew that breast cancer treatment would affect my *toes?* You don't know any of these details till you live through them—not from all the books of advice in the world. Cancer treatment is a spin of the roulette wheel. If my heart scans had not been good, with good ejection fractions, my chemo would have been stopped. Cancer can kill you but a stopped heart is a definite deal-breaker.

Yet I've made it through till today …. My friend Barbara, who comes to the infusion center for treatment of her MS and knows it's my last day there, shows up in the waiting room with a big box of cupcakes—we're having a party. These are the kind of cupcakes that have three inches of gooey icing on them and a little plastic football decoration as well.

A day to celebrate! Though Barbara is in a wheelchair, her husband guides her around the waiting room so she can offer cupcakes to everyone. The waiting room is a friendly place. There's coffee and hot chocolate and tea available, there's the ubiquitous TV (but not too loud), and there's conversation.

We talk about cannabis. Barbara and I both know cancer patients who take medical marijuana for their discomfort. The process does not evolve from the medical establishment—Dr. B did not recommend me for the substance, in fact she never once suggested it. The deal is done by going first to a "marijuana doctor" in the city. You are asked to carry with you some records of your disease. The illness does not have to be cancer, in particular. I discover the following:

> According to the Compassionate Use Act of 1996,
> seriously ill Californians have the right to obtain and use
> Marijuana—aka Cannabis—for medical purposes where
> the medical use is deemed appropriate and has been
> recommended by a physician who has determined that the
> person's health would benefit from the use of marijuana
> in the treatment of cancer, anorexia, AIDS, chronic pain,
> spasticity, glaucoma, arthritis, migraine, or any other
> illness for which marijuana provides relief.

You simply tell the doctor about your level of pain, or inability to sleep. He charges you a hundred dollars and gives you a letter to take to the marijuana dispensary. There you may choose the form of the drug that appeals to you. And what an array is available! If you don't want to smoke it, you can have chewy Dixie rolls shaped like Tootsie Rolls; you can have fruit lozenges, chocolate truffles, tinctures that go into your tea with a little milk or cream, crispy rice squares, and lifesavers that go below your tongue ("wintergreen flavor") for fast relief from pain.

I wonder why I didn't know all this when I was in the throes of the worst of the chemo treatment, when I was in the hospital, when I was throwing up at the 7-Eleven.

But today, I'm happy to have my cupcake, sweet and gooey and full of chemicals and white flour and shortening and the great monster itself: sugar.

There's an old gentleman in the waiting room with us; he's been listening to our conversation and smiling. Suddenly he offers me … a pen! I'm astonished because of the beauty of the pen, a pen enclosed by the most beautiful covering of elegant polished wood. This man cannot know I am obsessed with pens (pens and typewriters), that I am a writer, and that any pen is a treasure to me. I have never in my life passed a pen in the grass or the gutter that I didn't pick up and take home. I don't know what else to do but take the pen from his hand and exclaim with awe over its beauty.

He then unrolls a cloth and lays other pens out for us to see.

They're all just beautiful.

"I make them in my spare time," he says, smiling. "When I'm not here for chemo."

I thank him for showing me his pens—and offer back the one he gave to me. But no, "It's for you," he says. He's giving it to me for having lived through chemo. He's giving me a present of a pen.

"Maybe I'll write a book with it," I half-promise him, half-promise myself. But I don't think I will ever write about cancer. Who would want to relive these days?

Not me. Not ever.

When my infusion is over, I say my goodbye to all my old friends, my dear nurse Cristina, and Jesse, and Ivan and Cassandra (who empties the trash each time I'm there) and all the sweet chemo-pharmacists who walk by and talk to the patients, especially to one who was about to marry when I first met her, during my first chemo, and now is perhaps six months pregnant and glowing. What significant days of our lives we have all shared, we in the cancer ward.

I stop off to say goodbye to Dr. B. She and I are not parting by any means—we have dates every three months for the next five years. But today I have to give her the painting I did for her. I find her in the hall and give her the gift. She laughs at my amazing (my primitive!) artwork, and we ask a nurse to take our picture together.

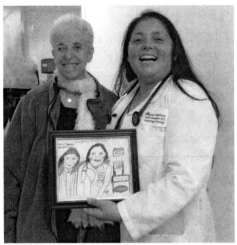

Merrill and Dr. B and painting

When I get home, I pull off my last chemo ID bracelet and drop it in a basket with all the others. That's it. Goodbye chemo jewelry. Goodbye for good.

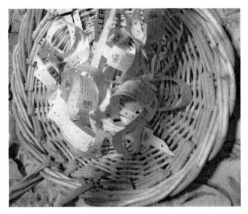

Basket of chemo bracelets

THIRTY-FIVE
PAINT THE SKY BLUE

THOUGH THERE ARE MANY CLASSES OFFERED at the Cancer Support Center, most of them deal with the agonies of cancer treatment. They offer advice on coping, talks on death and finances and meditation and chemo brain, information on robotic surgery, and when there is no longer hope, on hospice care. One class promises to be free of anxiety. "Watercolor Painting Class: bring a pen, a pencil, watercolor brushes, watercolor paper, watercolor paint, a palette, a rag, a sponge and a cup of water."

My friends and I have finished active cancer treatment, so we have technically "graduated" from our support group. A new group has formed to meet on the night we met but now there is a new facilitator; new people are facing the long road of treatment. In their group, as in ours, there will no doubt be some who will not graduate, but will die.

But we survivors miss one another. We long to see one another again. We send emails. We share pictures of pretty flowers and pets. We send political messages (a president is being elected). We live far from one another but not far from the cancer center.

"Let's become painters," one of us suggests. "Let's take the watercolor class. We can be together every Thursday morning and never once discuss disease!"

I always wondered if I had any talent to paint. I sometimes tried to draw a picture.

Once, in Siena, Italy, waiting for Joe to arrive and meet me for lunch, I sat in the piazza and drew the church I saw in front of me. But we were in Italy then, in the land of amazements of art, in the land of Botticelli. In Florence was the Duomo, the David. I knew nothing of the artist's life.

So why, with fingers that know mainly how to type, would I put a paintbrush in them? As to making images, I have a camera. I take pictures. My grandchildren hide their faces when they see me coming.

But the call of the support center draws me back; I want to be there with my fellow travelers, we who have shared this unexpected, treacherous journey. We, who started out as strangers, but who, at the end of our months together, now kiss one another hello and goodbye.

Joe and I go to the local crafts store to buy paints, palettes, brushes, and watercolor paper. Joe and some of his friends from the Caretaker's Group are also going to join the watercolor class. An adventure! A challenge. Something new to do and think about.

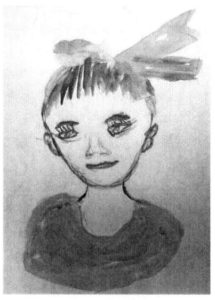

Merrill's painting of granddaughter in pink ribbon

Richard, our teacher, suggests that we paint an image he projects on a screen or simply an image we love from a photograph. In my wallet I have a picture of my granddaughter at her ballet class. I paint a rendition of her beautiful little face.

Clearly, the Italian greats have no reason to worry. Here is no spectacular talent bursting forth upon the universe. On another day, Richard projects a winter scene of a mountain range, trees, sky, a cloud or two. Again I ignore the recommended model and instead draw a picture of my house in Brooklyn, a recollection of a photo I have always loved: the house where I grew up, my aunt sitting on the windowsill of an upper story, washing the window, and my grandmother at another window, looking out at the street. To recreate this, I simply draw the standard shape of a house that children learn and put everyone I love at a window—myself, my aunt and grandmother, my sister, my doll, my mother and father, even my dog and my cat.

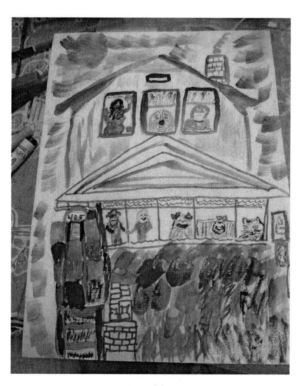

House in Brooklyn painting

This is exciting. Suddenly I am able to put myself back in time, into my childhood home, among the people who are all dead, except my sister, and here I am, by my own hand, living with them again, hearing their voices and seeing their smiles. I give them smiles even though I know far too well how much unhappiness swirled in that house.

This is a revelation for me. At home, on the dining room table, I set up my art studio. One meeting a week at the cancer center is not enough. I begin to draw and paint every day, almost always from photos that I discover in old boxes and albums. Though, as a writer, I have rendered so many of these memories in my stories and novels. Now, here I am, given a chance to relive them once again and this time transform them into a world of beauty and love—without stress, without loss, without death.

Again I recognize that I have come through the black days of cancer into a new kind of light and celebration. Who could have guessed?

THIRTY-SIX
INVITATION TO THE DANCE

IN MY BEDROOM, SOMETHING FALLS DOWN from a shelf in the
closet. There is my belly-dance costume from my long-ago life:
the fringed bikini top, the bejeweled skirt that hung lightly on my
hips (belly button visible, of course), the coin belt swinging and
still jingling as I hold up the shimmery cloth. The veil is there
too, gauzy, pink shading to purple, the gold snake bracelet for my
upper arm, and the pair of zills—those tiny cymbals belly dancers
wear upon their fingers to accompany the drummers and oud
players with their special rhythms.

Forty years ago I took my three little girls to the community
center so they could learn how to make origami swans. As I left
them in the classroom, I heard a low, thrumming drumbeat
with a rhythmic accompaniment of metallic clicks coming from
behind the closed doors of another room. The high wail of some
exotic instrument filled the hallway. I pushed open the door and
went in. A circle of women, clothed in swaths of chiffon, turned
and swirled on the carpeted floor of the big room. Gold coins
clicked and danced on their bellies, on their breasts, even on their
foreheads. Gold circles on their fingers flew like lightning to convey
an insistent signal to their arching bare feet and moving toes. The
teacher wore a red jewel in her navel. She shimmied her hips; she
did a spectacular backbend, her long dark hair brushing the floor.

Her drummer was a man with wavy brown hair; he wore a tan silk shirt, brown suede pants, and high leather boots. He played on a drum, a large pottery jug with a tight animal skin stretched across it. The teacher swayed and moved on her bare toes, undulating and twisting her upper body like a snake, leaning and hip-lifting her way forward till she had moved herself directly in front of the drummer and was dancing in place, her coins swinging and brushing his leather-clad knees. He never smiled and she never smiled, but their eyes held, not six inches apart, as she worked her amazing muscles into a wild and desperate shimmy. (He wasn't only her drummer; I could see that at once.)

I joined the class that very day. Each week, as my children made origami creatures, I learned the beauty of belly dance. The teacher, named Nefertiti, told me I had the rare gift of being "a natural." I practiced at home. My children were embarrassed, but at night in our bedroom, my husband was astonished and thrilled.

Will this costume still fit me? I lost so much weight during chemo, it is quite possible. Why not try it on? I close the bedroom door. I fasten the bikini top over my breasts. I pull the skirt over my hips, position the veil over my shoulders. I even slide the zills on the first and third fingers of each hand.

One day, in watercolor class, I do a painting of a belly dancer, which later I used on the cover of the ebook version of my novel *The Lady with the Moving Parts.*

I tentatively try the figure eights I remember from that long ago class and I do a few hip-lifts, but when I try to move myself across the floor in the remembered sinuous steps, my feet freeze as if an emergency brake has been thrown.

My frozen toes! They aren't getting the instructions from my brain. They are jammed on the carpet, little stubs of inanimate matter, innocent victims of chemotherapy.

I send a note to my oncologist and she refers me to a neurologist. He promptly sets me up for an electromyography and nerve conduction study. A cheerful, amiable man, he makes jokes as he sends shocks through my legs and inserts needles into my limbs, making my feet fly up through the air. A machine measures my responses. Is it painful? I barely pay attention. I feel calm and unthreatened. I already know the doctor's conclusion: *"Evaluation of a 74-year-old, right-handed woman complaining of numbness in her toes: The patient has bilateral sural neuropathy."* Numb toes. I could have saved us all the trouble.

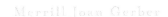

THE LADY WITH THE MOVING PARTS

Merrill Joan Gerber

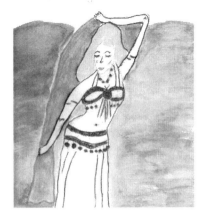

Belly dance painting

But without my sensitive toes, I will have to pack up my belly dance gear and put it into the closet. Another page torn from the book of life, another casualty of cancer. Yet, when a flyer comes from the Cancer Support Group for the Hoedown, I see one more chance to dance.

I often ponder why my husband, totally in tune with the rhythms of music, is a hippopotamus when it comes to dancing. Sometimes at home, when the moment is right, when the public TV station is playing Doo-wop music from the fifties, when the favorite song from my teens is being sung, I put my arms around Joe and we sway (usually in the kitchen) to the throbbing notes of "Hold Me, Thrill Me, Kiss Me." I sing into his ear along with the TV singers. I love the line that says, when he holds me in his arms he drives me slowly out of my mind. He is not really up for too much romance.

After five minutes of this, Joe disentangles my arms from around his neck and excuses himself to go either to his piano or his computer. I tell him many times how sexy dancing is, how I'd love for him to take me to some dark bar (not that we ever go to bars) and hold me in his arms and drive me slowly out of my mind. He simply doesn't get it. He will never get it. Men and women come from different planets. It's a known fact. But Joe does agree to go to the Hoedown. We cheerfully sit with other cancer patients and their families at the dinner tables set with Western decorations and colorful hats. We listen with pleasure to the music; we eat the barbecued ribs and chicken. (What! No plant-based food on this night?) There is live square dance music. A caller calls the steps. A member of the Cancer Support Center comes spinning by. She holds her arms out to me and pulls me up from my chair into the dance. We do-si-do, we hook our elbows and fly around in a circle, we skip up and down the line as others clap, we gasp for air and laugh.

My, do we have fun. Fun is a miracle we must revere, we who know all too well there can still be trouble up ahead. Fun means living. Fun can never be refused if it is offered. Here we are with our cancer friends at this great Hoedown of Life, all of us, who after great bouts of sighing and crying, are at last dancing, dancing, dancing.

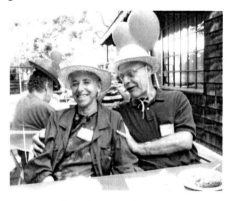

Merrill and Joe at the Hoedown

MERRILL JOAN GERBER is a prize-winning novelist and short story writer who has published ten novels—among them *King of The World*, which won the Pushcart Press Editors' Book Award for "an important and unusual book of literary distinction," and *The Kingdom of Brooklyn*, winner of the Ribalow Award from Hadassah Magazine for "the best English-language book of fiction on a Jewish theme"—as well as seven volumes of short stories, nine young-adult novels, and three books of non-fiction. Her short fiction has appeared in the *New Yorker*, the *Atlantic*, *Mademoiselle*, *Ladies' Home Journal*, and *Good Housekeeping*. *Redbook* magazine published forty-two of her stories, a record for any author. She has also published in literary journals such as the *Sewanee Review*, *Prairie Schooner*, *Shenandoah*, *Salmagundi*, the *Chattahoochee Review* and the *Virginia Quarterly Review*. Her story, "I Don't Believe This," won an O. Henry Prize. She has published essays in *Commentary*, the *Sewanee Review*, and the *Writer*. She earned her MA in English from Brandeis University and was awarded a Wallace Stegner Fiction Fellowship to Stanford University. She presently teaches fiction writing at the California Institute of Technology in Pasadena, California.

For more information, go to www.merrilljoangerber.com.

ALSO BY MERRILL JOAN GERBER

NOVELS
The Hysterectomy Waltz
The Victory Gardens of Brooklyn
Glimmering Girls: A Novel of the Fifties
Anna in the Afterlife
The Kingdom of Brooklyn
King of the World
The Lady With the Moving Parts
Now Molly Knows
An Antique Man
You Are Always Safe With Me

STORIES
This Is a Voice From Your Past: New and Selected Stories
Anna in Chains
This Old Heart of Mine: The Best of Merrill Joan Gerber's Redbook Stories
Honeymoon
Chattering Man: Stories and a Novella
Stop Here, My Friend

NON-FICTION
Gut Feelings: A Writer's Truths and Minute Inventions
Botticelli Blue Skies: An American in Florence
Old Mother, Little Cat: A Writer's Reflections on Her Kitten, Her Aged Mother,
and Life

YOUNG ADULT
Please Don't Kiss Me Now
Name a Star For Me
I'm Kissing as Fast as I Can
The Summer of My Indian Prince
Also Known as Sadzia, The Belly Dancer!
Marry Me Tomorrow
Even Pretty Girls Cry At Night
I'd Rather Think About Robby
Handsome as Anything

CPSIA information can be obtained
at www.ICGtesting.com
Printed in the USA
FSOW01n0014140916
24924FS

9 781603 815260